Basic Urogynaecology

Linda Cardozo
Consultant Obstetrician and Gynaecologist,
King's College Hospital,
London

Alfred Cutner
Registrar in Obstetrics and Gynaecology,
King's College Hospital Rotation,
London

Brian Wise
Research Registrar,
King's College Hospital,
London

Oxford   New York   Tokyo
OXFORD UNIVERSITY PRESS
1993

Oxford University Press, Walton Street, Oxford OX2 6DP

Oxford New York Toronto
Delhi Bombay Calcutta Madras Karachi
Kuala Lumpur Singapore Hong Kong Tokyo
Nairobi Dar es Salaam Cape Town
Melbourne Auckland Madrid
and associated companies in
Berlin Ibadan

Oxford is a trade mark of Oxford University Press

Published in the United States
by Oxford University Press Inc., New York

A catalogue record for this book is available from the British Library

Library of Congress Cataloging in Publication Data
Cardozo, Linda.
Basic urogynaecology / Linda Cardozo, Alfred Cutner, Brian Wise.
(Oxford medical publications)
Includes bibliographical references and index.
1. Urinary incontinence. 2. Urogynecology. 3. Generative organs,
Female—Diseases. I. Cutner, Alfred. II. Wise, Brian.
III. Title. IV. Series.
[DNLM: 1. Urinary Incontinence—diagnosis. 2. Urinary
Incontinence—therapy. WJ 146 C268b]
RC921.I5C37 1993 616.6'3—dc20 92-48233
ISBN 0-19-262360-5 (H'bk) ISBN 0-19-262359-1 (p'bk)

Typeset by Downdell, Oxford
Printed in Great Britain by
Dotesios Limited
Trowbridge, Wilts

Preface

Urinary incontinence is a condition which affects the lives of large numbers of men and women worldwide. Although rarely life threatening, it adversely affects the quality of life, causing disability and distress for the individual and significant morbidity within society. Until recently, little attention had been focused on this problem. In North America, however, the National Institutes of Health have realized that urinary incontinence is not only abnormal and antisocial but also extremely expensive, costing more than $12bn each year. They have called for a major research initiative to improve assessment and treatment of Americans with urinary incontinence.

Urinary incontinence affects the social, psychological, occupational, domestic, physical, and sexual aspects of life for 15 to 30 per cent of women in all age groups. Sufferers may have to give up many of their usual routines, with obvious detriment to social interactions, relationships, careers, and psychological well-being. Normal activities such as travelling, household chores, physical recreation, and hobbies are all severely restricted. A way of life arranged around the location of toilets and avoidance of potentially embarrassing situations may develop, leading to social isolation and diminished self-esteem. Marital harmony is impaired, partly because of the adverse effect on sexual relationships and the lack of understanding of the condition. Many women try to hide the problem from everyone including their spouse because of the shame they feel.

Before the 1970s, the aetiology of urinary incontinence was poorly understood and classification was vague. Treatment was haphazard with poor long-term results. This led to disenchantment amongst women and doctors and an unfortunate attitude of acceptance developed. It was only with the advent of uro-dynamic studies, some twenty years ago, that the outlook for women with urinary incontinence improved considerably. Unfortunately, the correlation between clinical diagnosis and urodynamic diagnosis is poor and, as the appropriate treatment for the various conditions is completely different, it is important to make an accurate diagnosis before treatment is commenced.

Much can be done to alleviate the problem of urinary incontinence. Treatment ranges from the very simple, such as habit re-training, right through to complex surgical procedures. Although it is not possible to cure everyone, something can always be done to improve the situation, even if it is only the provision of pads, pants, and incontinence aids or advice from the local continence adviser.

This book is designed to help all those who are interested in urinary problems in women. It is deliberately written in a didactic style with only a few key references from the literature. However, further suggested reading is included at the end of the book for those who wish to delve deeper into this important subject.

London   L.C.
July 1992   A.C.
                                                     B.G.W.

Foreword

STUART L. STANTON, FRCS, FRCOG
Consultant Gynaecologist and Urogynaecologist, St George's Hospital, London

The last twenty years have seen incontinence become a respectable condition, both for the patient to admit to and for the clinician to make it a lifetime interest. Urodynamics has become a valued science and urogynaecology an accepted branch of gynaecology, both in the United Kingdom and further afield. The serious training of urogynaecologists has commenced and in this, the Royal College of Obstetricians and Gynaecologists has taken an important lead. Our nursing colleagues in the UKCC have encouraged specialization by establishing the role of continence nurse advisors and many professional and patient organizations have been founded to facilitate communication of research and clinical issues.

There has been a steady burgeoning of books on the subject: there were two or three in the early 1970s and there are at least thirty currently available, some in their second and third editions. Is there room for one more? An unqualified yes.

Linda Cardozo is the first of a new generation of urogynaecologists specifically qualified in this area, and has in turn stimulated others, such as her co-authors Alfred Cutner and Brian Wise, to follow her. They are both her research fellows at Kings College Hospital and, together with Linda Cardozo, have successfully produced an eminently readable and clear book on urogynaecology. Its concise and direct style is consistent throughout the book, which covers all the topics included in urogynaecology. It is a mix of conventional subjects and the more practical management orientated topics—features which will appeal to the urogynaecologist in training, the general gynaecologists, the general practitioner, and to the more discriminating senior medical student.

The chapters are well written and the book has a clinical and practical balance, which most of its competitors have failed to achieve. It is well illustrated and compactly referenced. I am pleased to wish it a very great success.

Contents

Contents

I

Background

1

Embryology, anatomy, physiology, and pharmacology

INTRODUCTION

The lower urinary tract comprises the bladder and urethra which, in association with supporting ligaments and muscles, act as a single functional unit (Fig. 1.1).

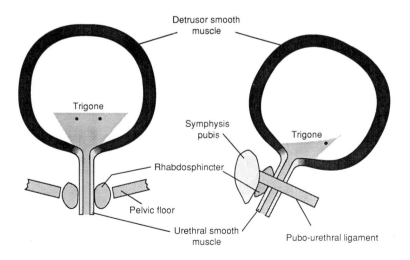

Fig. 1.1 Anatomy of the lower urinary tract.

EMBRYOLOGY

The developing embryo initially consists of a bilaminar structure containing ectoderm and endoderm which subsequently become separated by the mesoderm (Fig. 1.2). The yolk sac is lined by

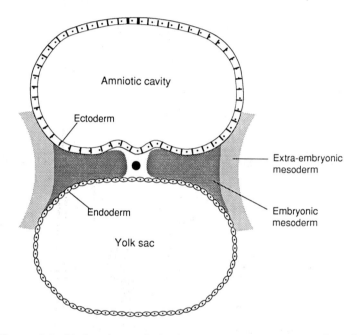

Figure 1.2 Embryology of the lower urinary tract: a 17-day old embryo.

endoderm and part of this becomes invaginated into the embryo to form the gut (Fig. 1.3). A diverticulum develops from the hindgut which is known as the allantois (Fig. 1.4). That part of the hindgut which is connected to the allantois is called the cloaca. Division of the cloaca by a wedge of mesenchymal tissue called the urorectal septum results in the formation of an anterior

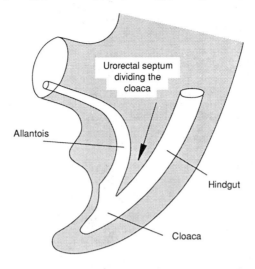

Fig. 1.3 Embryology of the lower urinary tract: a four-week old embryo.

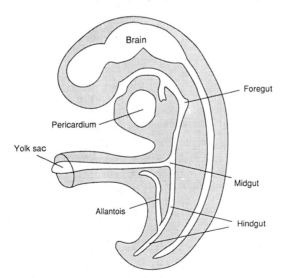

Fig. 1.4 Embryology of the lower urinary tract: a five-week old embryo.

part (the primitive bladder) and a posterior part (the anorectal canal) (Fig. 1.5).

At the same time, the kidneys are developing in the mesenchymal tissue. The first stage is the pronephros, but this subsequently disappears. The mesonephros develops from mesenchymal tissue and on each side its tubules open into a single collecting duct known as the mesonephric duct. The mesonephros functions initially as a primitive kidney but subsequently undergoes degeneration. The mesonephric duct develops an outgrowth, the ureteric bud, which will become the ureter. The distal end of the mesonephric duct enters the anterior part of the cloaca, on each side. That part of the primitive bladder above this point is the definitive bladder and the part below is the urogenital sinus (Fig. 1.5).

The caudal part of the mesonephric duct is absorbed by the bladder, thus drawing in the ureteric duct. With growth of the bladder the ureteric ducts move laterally and the mesonephric ducts come to lie more caudally, close together at that part of the primitive bladder which will become the urethra. The area of the bladder derived from the mesonephric ducts will become the trigone (Fig. 1.6).

Thus the upper part of the bladder is derived from the yolk sac and lined by endoderm, and the trigone, derived from the mesonephric ducts, is lined by cells of mesodermal origin. It is generally believed that the trigonal surface is later replaced by cells of endodermal origin.

The most caudal part of the cloaca is called the urogenital sinus and this forms the distal part of the urethra and vagina in the female. The fallopian tubes, uterus, and cervix are formed from the paramesonephric ducts which are an invagination of coelomic epithelium which is of mesodermal origin. Thus the fallopian tubes, uterus, and trigone appear to have a common embryological origin and the upper bladder and lower part of the urethra and vagina another. Full development occurs by the twelfth week of intrauterine life (Moore 1988).

Embryology, anatomy, physiology, and pharmacology 7

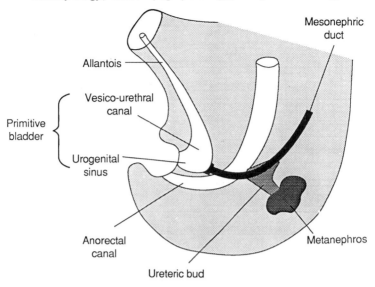

Fig. 1.5 Embryology of the lower urinary tract: a six-week old embryo.

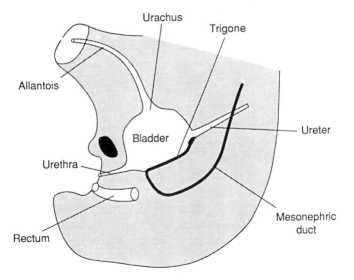

Fig. 1.6 Embryology of the lower urinary tract: an eight-week old embryo.

ANATOMY

The lower urinary tract is lined by transitional-cell epithelium.
The wall of the bladder is composed of a syncytium of smooth
muscle fibres known as the detrusor. Contraction of this mesh-
work of fibres results in simultaneous reduction of the bladder
in all its dimensions. The triangular area of the bladder bounded
by the two ureteric orifices and the proximal part of the urethra
is known as the trigone. The smooth muscle of the trigone has
two layers. It is less developed than the detrusor which extends
behind it.

The female urethra is about 4–5 cm long. At the bladder neck
there is smooth muscle which is generally believed to be a distinct
entity consisting of an inner longitudinal and outer oblique
layer. It is not thought to be functionally important in the female
although it may play a small role in bladder-neck opening.

The urethral sphincter can be divided into intrinsic and
extrinsic portions (Gosling and Dixon 1979) (Fig. 1.7). The
intrinsic part consists of epithelial, vascular, connective tissue,
and muscular elements (Rud *et al.* 1980). The rhabdosphincter is
a circular ring of striated muscle. It is thickest anteriorly, thins
laterally, and is virtually absent posteriorly. The muscle contains
mainly slow-twitch fibres which are able to contract over long
periods of time without fatigue. This is important in the maintenance of continence at rest.

The extrinsic sphincter mechanism comprises the striated
muscle of the levator ani through which the urethra passes. Its
fibres run laterally to the urethra, just inferior to the rhabdosphincter. The fibres are mainly of the fast-twitch type and are
therefore able to contract more efficiently but over shorter
periods of time. This is important during periods of exertion.

The bladder neck is supported in the correct position by the
connective-tissue supports. These are known as the pubovesical
or pubourethral ligaments (DeLancey 1989). They appear to

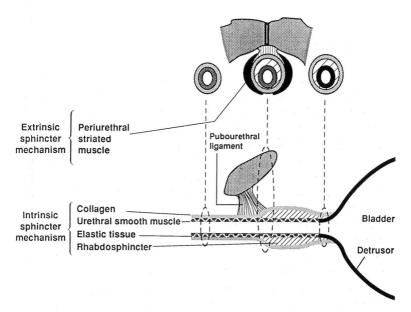

Fig. 1.7 Anatomy of the urethral sphincter mechanism.

have both passive and active function: supporting the bladder neck in the correct position and also causing opening of the bladder neck on initiation of micturition. These supports maintain the proximal two-thirds of the urethra in an intra-abdominal position.

The urethra is lined by transitional-cell epithelium but distally the lining becomes stratified squamous epithelium. The submucosa contains venous plexuses which contribute to urethral resistance and help it to form a watertight seal. However, there are conflicting opinions regarding the importance of these venous plexuses in the maintenance of continence. They are thought to contribute one-third of the urethral pressure and may therefore be important in the development of genuine stress incontinence in post-menopausal women.

INNERVATION

The bladder normally has a capacity of 400–600 ml and is capable of expanding to accommodate this large volume for a small increase in pressure. The innervation of the lower urinary tract is summarized by Khanna (1986). The main innervation of the detrusor is parasympathetic, which causes contraction. There is also β-sympathetic innervation which results in relaxation. The urethral smooth muscle is innervated by α-sympathomimetics which cause contraction. However, this is an over-simplification of lower urinary tract innervation as there appears to be overlap of receptors and interaction between parasympathetic and sympathetic actions.

The rhabdosphincter and levator ani are supplied by somatic nerves derived from sacral roots (S2 to S4). The fibres to the rhabdosphincter travel via the pelvic splanchnics whereas those to the levator ani travel via the perineal branch of the pudendal nerve.

Visceral afferent fibres travel with the thoraco-lumbar and sacral efferent nerves conveying the sensation of bladder distension. The central nervous control of micturition is complex and requires a sacral spinal reflex controlled by the cerebral cortex, the cerebellum, and subcortical areas including the thalamus, basal ganglia, limbic system, hypothalamus, and pontine reticular formation.

There are parasympathetic, sympathetic and somatic afferent and efferent connections from the brain stem. This visceral reflex is controlled by both excitatory and inhibitory centres which under normal circumstances prevent detrusor contractions and maintain urethral sphincter control, thereby inhibiting micturition. It would appear that the sympathetic innervation together with their thoraco-lumbar afferents are concerned mainly with the filling and storage phases of the micturition cycle whereas the parasympathetic innervation and its afferents are concerned with normal voiding. The innervation of the lower urinary tract is shown in Fig. 1.8.

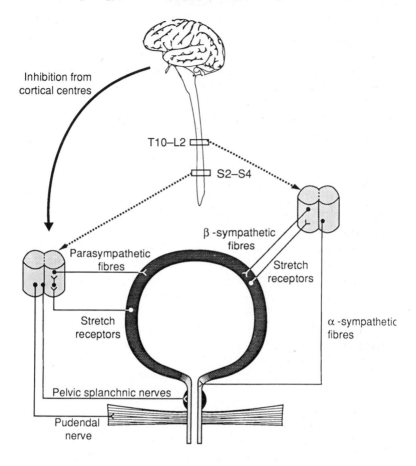

Inhibition from
cortical centres

T10–L2

S2–S4

β -sympathetic
fibres

Parasympathetic
fibres

Stretch
receptors

Stretch
receptors

α -sympathetic
fibres

Pelvic splanchnic nerves

Pudendal
nerve

Fig. 1.8   Innervation of the lower urinary tract.

PHYSIOLOGY

Filling phase

Urine produced by the kidneys enters the bladder via the ureters
at 0.5–5 ml per minute. During filling the detrusor remains

relaxed, allowing the bladder to fill without any significant rise
in pressure. This is due to cortical inhibition of reflex arcs acting
on the detrusor. Continence is maintained by occlusive forces
acting on the urethra. The rhabdosphincter remains contracted
and, in addition, the urethral epithelium forms folds, resulting
in a watertight seal.

Storage phase

During periods of exertion, increased intra-abdominal pressure
is transmitted to the bladder, which tends to cause expulsion of
urine. However, the upper two-thirds of the urethra is normally
supported in an intra-abdominal position by the pubourethral
ligaments, and the sphincter mechanism (especially the extrinsic
part) exerts additional force. The increased pressure is also
transmitted to the bladder neck and proximal urethra, thus
maintaining continence. This is known as the positive closure
pressure.

Voiding phase

At an appropriate time voiding is initiated. There is inhibition of
sympathetic activity resulting in urethral relaxation and, in
addition, voluntary relaxation of the rhabdosphincter and
levator ani. Following this, inhibition of the voiding reflex arc
by cortical centres is suppressed and the detrusor starts to
contract due to parasympathetic activity (Tanagho and Miller
1970). After voiding has been completed, the rhabdosphincter
contracts, as does the pelvic floor, and there is once again
cortical inhibition resulting in detrusor relaxation.

   Continence is a learnt phenomenon which depends on intact
nerve pathways combined with normal lower urinary tract
morphology. At rest it depends on bladder compliance, intact
neurological pathways, and an effective intrinsic sphincter
mechanism. During exertion, the correct position of the proximal urethra, the extrinsic urethral sphincter mechanism, and
the state of the urethral mucosa are important factors. Appro-

priate voiding relies on voluntary relaxation of the urethral sphincter accompanied by removal of cortical inhibition.

Although innervation is well documented, other substances are known to influence lower urinary tract function possibly through further modification of receptor function. Suggested transmitters include PGE_2 (prostaglandin E_2), $PGF_{2\alpha}$ (prostaglandin $F_{2\alpha}$), calcitonin-gene-related peptide (CGRP), substance P, and vasoactive intestinal polypeptide (VIP).

HORMONAL INFLUENCES

In addition to parasympathetic and sympathetic effects and their modification by prostaglandins and neuropeptides, steroid hormones will further influence lower urinary tract function (Miodrag *et al.* 1988).

Oestrogen has been shown to enhance detrusor cholinergic action and urethral α-adrenergic action. Progesterone is thought to enhance detrusor β-adrenergic action. Apart from affecting lower urinary tract responses to adrenergic and cholinergic activity, oestrogen may affect lower urinary tract function in a more indirect manner.

Urethral function relies on its epithelial lining, vascularity, and supporting connective tissue. The epithelium lining of the trigone and urethra alter in response to oestrogen status and the submucosal vasculature is also oestrogen dependent.

Collagen is formed by fibroblasts whose activity is oestrogen dependent. The effects of oestrogen are of more importance in low oestrogen states, which occur post-menopausally where oestrogen therapy has been shown to improve lower urinary tract symptomatology.

Thus the function of the lower urinary tract is complex and involves the interaction of not only the parasympathetic and sympathetic nerves but also neuropeptides and steroid hormones. Any imbalance in this system can lead to lower urinary tract dysfunction or incontinence.

PHARMACOLOGY

Drugs affecting the lower urinary tract can exert their influence either directly on neurological pathways or indirectly through mediators (Wein 1986). Only those of clinical importance will be discussed. These are shown in Table 1.1.

Table 1.1   Pharmacology of the lower urinary tract

	Effect on detrusor contractility	Effect on urethral resistance
Anticholinergic activity	−	
Cholinergic activity	+	
Calcium-channel blockers	−	
β-Agonists	−	
α-Agonists	(+)	+
α-Antagonists	(−)	−
Skeletal-muscle relaxants	(−)	−
Central nervous system depressants	−	

Drugs can alter detrusor contractility by affecting the action of acetylcholine. Any drugs with anticholinergic properties inhibit detrusor contractions, and cholinergic agents will promote bladder emptying by enhancing detrusor contraction. Calcium is necessary for muscle contractility and therefore calcium-channel blockers will inhibit detrusor contractions. The detrusor also has some sympathetic innervation which is mainly of the β-sympathetic type. β-Sympathetic agonists will inhibit detrusor contractions slightly. Drugs with α-antagonistic properties decrease detrusor contractility whereas α-agonists may slightly increase detrusor contractility. In addition to these, skeletal-muscle relaxants, central nervous system depressants, and narcotic agents all reduce detrusor contractility.

Urethral innervation is mainly α-sympathetic and drugs which affect this activity will alter urethral resistance. Drugs with α-sympathetic activity increase urethral resistance and α-antagonists do the reverse. In addition, skeletal-muscle relaxants decrease urethral resistance.

The effects of hormones on the lower urinary tract are indirect and have already been described. The actual effect that a particular agent has on the lower urinary tract is determined by its relative parasympathetic and sympathetic properties, either agonistic or antagonistic, and is further modified by its central nervous system activity.

REFERENCES

DeLancey, J.O.L. (1989). Pubovesical ligament: a separate structure from the urethral supports ('Pubo-Urethral Ligaments'). *Neurourology and Urodynamics*, **8**, 53–61.

Gosling, J.A. and Dixon, J. (1979). Light and electronmicroscopic observations on the human external urethral sphincter. *J. Anat.*, **129**, 216 (Abstract).

Khanna, O.M.P. (1986). Disorders of micturition: neurophysiological basis and results of drug therapy. *Urology*, **8**, 316–28.

Miodrag, A., Castleden, C.M., and Vallance, T.R. (1988). Sex hormones and the female lower urinary tract. *Drugs*, **36**, 491–504.

Moore, K.L. (1988). The urogenital system. In *The developing human. Clinically orientated embryology* (4th edn). Ch. 13, pp. 246–85. Saunders, Philadelphia.

Rud, T., Andersson, K.E., Asmussen, M., Hunting, A., and Ulsten, U. (1980). Factors maintaining the intraurethral pressure in women. *Invest. Urol.*, **17**, 343–7.

Tanagho, E.A. and Miller, E.R. (1970). Initiation of voiding. *Br. J. Urol.*, **42**, 175–83.

Wein, A.J. (1986). In *Surgery of female incontinence* (2nd edn) (ed. S.L. Stanton and E.A. Tanagho). pp. 229–45. Springer, Berlin.

2

Prevalence and pathophysiology of lower urinary tract disorders

INTRODUCTION

Incontinence is defined by the International Continence Society (ICS) as a condition in which there is involuntary leakage of urine, which is objectively demonstrable, and is a social or hygienic problem (Abrams *et al.* 1990). The ICS is a multidisciplinary association of urologists, gynaecologists, and basic scientists with a special interest in urinary incontinence. Throughout this book, all terms and definitions (see also the Appendix) conform to those defined by the ICS committee on standardization of terminology.

PREVALENCE

Urinary symptoms are very common in the healthy population and estimates of the prevalence of incontinence vary, depending on the sample of women investigated. In a large study, Thomas *et al.* (1980) showed a gradual increase in the prevalence of incontinence with age, such that approximately 40 per cent of women in their eighties suffer from the condition. Young women may also be affected, and in a study by Nemir and Middleton (1954), 52 per cent of nulliparous students complained of having been incontinent at some time. The prevalence of incontinence is greater in women attending their general practitioner or the gynaecology clinic than in the general population, where between 30 and 50 per cent may complain of incontinence.

The highest rates of incontinence are found in the geriatric and psychogeriatric populations, where more than 40 per cent and 90 per cent of patients respectively are incontinent.

In 1991 Market and Opinion Research International (MORI) were commissioned to conduct a survey on health by questionnaire, with particular reference to incontinence (MORI 1991). One in seven women admitted to having problems of incontinence at some time, and a third of these women were currently incontinent. From these figures alone it is estimated that there may be 2.5 million female sufferers nationwide. Over a third of women questioned knew a friend or relative with incontinence, so the overall prevalence may be far greater.

URINARY SYMPTOMS

Incontinence

There are different types of urinary incontinence, and these may be found in isolation or in combination. They are summarized in Table 2.1. **Stress incontinence** is the involuntary loss of urine which occurs upon raising intra-abdominal pressure, e.g. when coughing, sneezing, laughing, or during exercise. **Urge incontinence** is the involuntary loss of urine which is preceded by a sudden strong desire to void. **Dribble incontinence** implies the continual leakage of small volumes of urine. **Giggle incontinence**

Table 2.1 Patterns of incontinence

Stress	Caused by coughing, sneezing, exercise
Urge	Preceded by sudden, strong urge to void
Dribble	Constant
Giggle	Isolated symptom, <25 yrs
Intercourse	Caused by penetration, orgasm
Nocturnal enuresis	Leakage at night

is a specific type of incontinence which is confined to girls and young women (under 25 years old) and is often self-limiting. **Incontinence during intercourse** is a distressing condition and may occur during penetration or at the time of orgasm. **Nocturnal enuresis** is the term used to describe involuntary loss of urine during sleep. All these symptoms of urinary incontinence are common amongst women, but are abnormal.

Irritative symptoms

- Frequency.
- Nocturia.
- Urgency.
- Dysuria.

In addition to incontinence, many women complain of irritative symptoms. **Frequency** is generally considered to be seven or more voids during the day, and **nocturia** as awakening two or more times during the night in order to pass urine. **Urgency** is a sudden desire to void and may lead on to **urge incontinence**, with involuntary loss of urine occurring before the woman can reach the toilet. **Dysuria** involves the occurrence of pain on micturition.

Voiding difficulties

- Poor flow.
- Prolonged voiding.
- Straining to void.
- Incomplete emptying.
- Double micturition.

The subjective impression of difficulty in emptying the bladder is not uncommon in women. They may volunteer that they have a poor stream, and that their voiding time is prolonged. They may need to strain to improve the urinary flow, or may exert pressure suprapubically. Following voiding they may feel that the bladder is incompletely empty and need to void again within a few minutes.

THE CAUSES OF INCONTINENCE

Incontinence will occur whenever the intravesical pressure exceeds the urethral closure pressure (Enhorning 1961). Thus, uninhibited detrusor contractions, spontaneous relaxation of the urethral sphincter, or dysfunction of the urethral closure mechanisms may result in leakage. The various causes of incontinence are summarized below.

- Genuine stress incontinence.
- Detrusor instability.
- Overflow incontinence.
- Fistula.
- Congenital abnormality (e.g. ectopic ureter, epispadias).
- Temporary (e.g. immobility, faecal impaction, urinary tract infection).
- Functional (lack of voluntary control).
- Miscellaneous (e.g. urethral diverticulum).

Genuine stress incontinence

Definition   The involuntary loss of urine when intravesical pressure exceeds the maximum urethral closure pressure in the absence of detrusor activity.

Incidence   Commonest cause of incontinence in women. Demonstrated in 40–60 per cent of women investigated.

Pathophysiology   See Fig. 2.1.

Clinical features   Symptom of stress incontinence, which may be demonstrable on clinical examination.

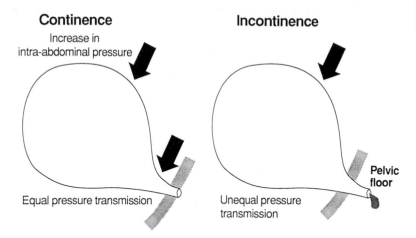

Continence   **Incontinence**

Increase in
intra-abdominal pressure

Equal pressure transmission   Unequal pressure
                                   transmission

Pelvic
floor

Fig. 2.1   Pathophysiology of genuine stress incontinence (GSI).

Aetiology and associated factors
- Multiparity—vaginal deliveries.
- Previous trauma to urethra (e.g. surgery, infection).
- Oestrogen deficiency.
- Raised intra-abdominal pressure.

Genuine stress incontinence (GSI) arises due to deficiency
in the urethral closure mechanisms during episodes of stress,
e.g. coughing, running, etc. Weakness of the rhabdosphincter
urethrae, levator ani muscles, and pubourethral ligaments predisposes to this condition. Maintenance of the bladder neck and
proximal urethra in an intra-abdominal position is an important
factor in the mechanism of continence. In this position, any rise
in intra-abdominal pressure will be transmitted equally to the
bladder neck and proximal urethra, thus maintaining the positive pressure gradient which normally exists between the urethra
and the bladder. Descent of the bladder neck will result in loss of
intra-abdominal pressure transmission to the proximal urethra
during stress, and incontinence occurs because bladder pressure
then exceeds the urethral closure pressure.

GSI is more common in multiparous women and may arise following denervation and reinnervation of the pelvic floor, which can occur following vaginal delivery (Smith *et al.* 1989). Damage to the supporting structures of the bladder and levator ani muscles leads to the association of GSI and prolapse, although the two conditions can exist independently. Impairment of the function of the urethral sphincter may arise following repeated trauma from surgery, instrumentation, or catheterization.

Fibrosis of the urethral mucosa may result from chronic inflammation leading to a functionless 'drainpipe urethra'. The integrity of the epithelium of the urethra is maintained by oestrogen, which increases vascularity and collagen content. The increased prevalence and exacerbation of existing GSI, which tends to occur in postmenopausal women, may in part be due to oestrogen deficiency.

Leakage of urine in women with genuine stress incontinence will be exacerbated by any condition that results in raised intra-abdominal pressure, e.g. chronic bronchitis, constipation, abdomino-pelvic mass, ascites.

Detrusor instability

Definition A condition in which the detrusor is objectively shown to contract, either spontaneously or on provocation, during bladder filling, while the subject is attempting to inhibit micturition. This is a urodynamic diagnosis made at the time of cystometry.

Incidence The second most common cause of female urinary incontinence. It is demonstrated in 20–40 per cent of referrals for urodynamic studies, but may be present in up to 10 per cent of the population, most of whom do not seek help.

Pathophysiology See Fig. 2.2.

Clinical features Symptoms of urgency, urge incontinence, frequency, nocturia, nocturnal enuresis. No specific physical signs.

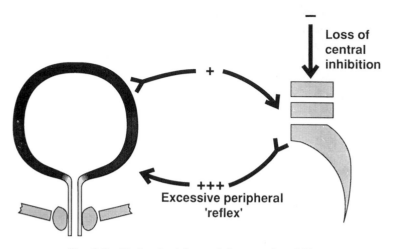

Fig. 2.2   Pathophysiology of detrusor instability.

Aetiology and associated factors

In the majority of cases no underlying cause is found for the condition and therefore the term 'idiopathic detrusor instability' is used. Poorly learnt bladder control as an infant may be the cause of detrusor instability in women with life-long symptoms, or maladaptive patterns of voiding may be adopted later in life. Less frequently, there is objective evidence of neurological disease, e.g. multiple sclerosis, upper motor neurone lesions due to spinal cord disruption. There is a small but definite incidence of detrusor instability arising *de novo* following pelvic surgery, especially after procedures for the treatment of incontinence. In men, detrusor instability may arise as a result of outflow obstruction due to prostatic hypertrophy, but the same association with outflow obstruction is not as evident in women.

Overflow incontinence

Definition   Incontinence occurs when bladder filling exceeds the functional bladder capacity. There is always an associated impairment of bladder sensation and/or the normal voiding mechanism.

Incidence   Common in the elderly, due to a hypotonic detrusor. Beware post-operatively.

Pathophysiology   See Fig. 2.3.

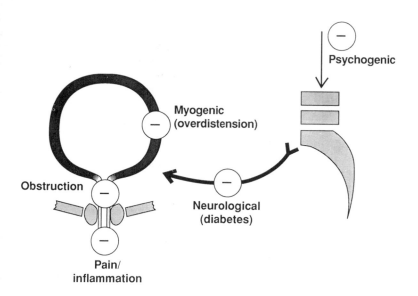

Fig. 2.3   Pathophysiology of voiding difficulties.

Clinical features   Symptoms of stress incontinence, frequency, recurrent urinary tract infections, or voiding difficulties. Enlarged, palpable bladder on examination.

Aetiology and associated factors
See Table 2.2.

Table 2.2 The causes of urinary retention

Neurological	Lower motor neurone lesion
	Peripheral neuropathy (Diabetes mellitus)
	Autonomic lesion
	Detrusor sphincter dyssynergia
	Local pain reflex
Myogenic injury	Overdistension
Pharmacological	Anticholinergic agents
	Tricyclic antidepressants
	α-Adrenergic agonists
	Epidural anaesthesia
	Ganglion blocking agents
Pain/inflammation	Postoperative/postpartum
	Herpes genitalis
	Bartholin abscess
	Acute urethritis
	Acute vulvovaginitis
Obstruction	Stricture
	Urethral oedema post-surgery
	Foreign body, e.g. calculus
	Impacted pelvic mass, e.g. fibroids
	Urethral kinking due to a cystocele
	Faecal impaction
Endocrine	Hypothyroidism
Psychogenic	Voluntary inhibition of micturition
	Dementia

Urinary fistula

Definition   A fistula is defined as an abnormal connection between two epithelial surfaces. It forms, in this case, between the urothelium of the ureter, bladder, or urethra, and the epithelium of the uterus or vagina. Sites of fistulae are shown in Fig. 2.4.

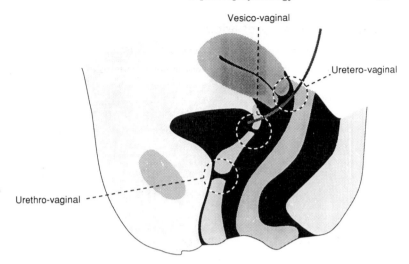

Fig. 2.4 Common sites of urinary fistulae.

Incidence Uncommon in the western world except post-operatively. More common in countries with poor obstetric facilities. Fistulae may occur in cases of advanced cervical malignancy or following radiotherapy.

Clinical features Continual incontinence which occurs both day and night. Site of fistula may be visible on speculum examination.

Aetiology and associated factors
The causes of urinary fistulae are summarized below.

- Surgical trauma (e.g. hysterectomy, Caesarean section, vaginal repair).
- Pelvic malignancy (e.g. direct invasion, post-radiotherapy).
- Obstetric (e.g. obstructed labour).

Worldwide, the most common cause of urinary fistula is obstructed labour secondary to cephalopelvic disproportion.

Such fistulae are caused by sloughing of bladder or urethral tissue due to ischaemia, following prolonged pressure. Infection is often a complicating factor in such cases. In the developed world, however, surgical trauma is the main cause of fistulae. The amount of tissue loss is less than for obstetric fistulae and superimposed infection less common. Advanced malignancy of the endometrium or cervix may result in direct spread of tumour into the bladder. More commonly fistula formation will follow treatment with radiotherapy, or after surgery to a previously irradiated pelvis.

Other causes of urinary incontinence

The conditions mentioned above account for the majority of cases of incontinence. However, the following may result in urinary symptoms including incontinence.

Urethral diverticulum

This may arise following trauma to the urethra, during childbirth, or following surgery, but more commonly as a result of acute infection of the genitourinary tract by *Chlamydia trachomatis* or *Neisseria gonorrhoeae*. Clinically, a diverticulum may present with symptoms of frequency, urgency, dysuria, urethral discomfort, or urethral discharge. The diverticulum may fill with urine during micturition and result in incontinence when the patient stands up.

Temporary causes of incontinence

The presence of a urinary tract infection (UTI) may result in incontinence in an otherwise healthy patient. Acute infection will also exacerbate any pre-existing urinary symptoms. Exclusion of a UTI is an essential initial step in the management of the incontinent patient.

In the elderly patient, reduced mobility and dexterity may be confounding factors that give rise to or worsen the problem of incontinence. Faecal impaction is a common cause of voiding difficulty and overflow incontinence in this age group.

REFERENCES

Abrams, P., Blaivas, J.G., Stanton, S.L., and Andersen, J.T. (1990). The standardisation of terminology of lower urinary tract function. *Br. J. Obstet. Gynaecol.* (Suppl.) **6**, 1–16.

Enhorning, G. (1961). Simultaneous recordings of the intravesical and intraurethral pressure. *Acta Chir. Scand.* (Suppl.) **276**, 1–68.

Market and Opinion Research International (1991). Health survey questionnaire. Topline results, 6040. MORI, 95 Southwark Street, London SE5 0HX, UK.

Nemir, A. and Middleton, R.P. (1954). Stress incontinence in young nulliparous women—a statistical study. *Am. J. Obstet. Gynecol.*, **68**, 1166–8.

Smith, A.R.B., Hosker, G.L., and Warrell, D.W. (1989). The role of pudendal nerve damage in the aetiology of genuine stress incontinence in women. *Br. J. Obstet. Gynaecol.*, **96**, 29–32.

Thomas, T.M., Plymat, K.R., Blannin, J., and Meade, T.W. (1980). Prevalence of urinary incontinence. *Br. Med. J.*, **281**, 1243–5.

II

Making a diagnosis

3

History and examination

INTRODUCTION

Just as in all other areas of medicine, the path towards diagnosis begins with the taking of a comprehensive history. This should document all urinary symptoms, past medical and surgical problems, past gynaecological and obstetric history, any inter-current medical disorder, social and sexual history. A careful physical examination should then be carried out, after which the need for further investigation may be assessed.

UROLOGICAL HISTORY

Urinary symptoms are very common among women of all ages, and rarely occur in isolation. Each symptom, or symptom complex, may be caused by one or more different conditions, and so a diagnosis cannot be made solely on the basis of a history.

Most women will complain of incontinence in addition to other symptoms. The onset and duration of incontinence should be sought, although this is of little value in predicting the diagnosis. Many women will associate the onset of symptoms with pregnancy or delivery, following hysterectomy, the meno-pause, trauma or surgery to the lumbo-sacral spine, or the onset of neurological disease. Table 3.1 summarizes urinary symptoms and their causes.

Table 3.1 Urinary symptoms and their causes

Symptom	Possible underlying conditions
Frequency (Seven or more voids per day) **Nocturia** (Two or more voids per night) **Urgency**	**Gynaecological/urological** Detrusor instability Sensory urgency Urinary tract infection Cystocele Urinary residual Genuine stress incontinence Pregnancy Abdominal/pelvic mass Intravesical lesion Interstitial cystitis Small capacity bladder Radiation Menopause Urethral syndrome Urethral obstruction Urethral diverticulum Genitourinary infection **Psychological** Excessive fluid intake Habit Anxiety **Medical** Diuretics Diabetes mellitus Diabetes insipidus Congestive cardiac failure Neurological (detrusor hyperreflexia) Renal failure
Urge incontinence	Detrusor instability Sensory urgency Rarely urinary tract infection, intravesical lesion
Stress incontinence	Genuine stress incontinence Detrusor instability Retention with overflow

The degree of incontinence varies widely from the occasional loss of a few drops of urine to frequent episodes of complete bladder emptying.

The pattern of incontinence is important but not diagnostic. Women who complain solely of stress incontinence are likely to suffer from genuine stress incontinence, whereas women complaining of urge incontinence, urgency, frequency, and nocturia are more likely to have detrusor instability. The majority of women will have a mixture of symptoms of incontinence, irritative symptoms, and possibly symptoms of voiding difficulty. Table 3.2 gives important points in the urological history.

Table 3.2 Important points for a urological history

Incontinence	Onset
	Duration
	Degree
	Type
Irritative symptoms	Frequency
	Urgency
	Nocturia
	Dysuria
Voiding difficulty	Poor stream
	Prolonged voiding
	Straining
	Incomplete emptying
Urinary tract infection	(? Proven)
	Frequency
Others	Bedwetting as a child
	Previous catheterization
	Previous urinary retention
	Previous treatment

GYNAECOLOGICAL HISTORY

Many women may be suffering from other gynaecological disorders in addition to urinary incontinence. It is important to highlight these as they may be involved in the aetiology of the urinary symptoms, or their treatment may alter management of the bladder problem. In particular, symptoms of uterovaginal prolapse commonly coexist with urinary incontinence, although they are not always directly related in aetiology. A sexual history is important as coital incontinence, when present, will have an adverse effect on libido and satisfaction for both partners. Incontinence at orgasm is a distressing symptom occasionally found in women with detrusor instability. The exacerbation of urinary symptoms prior to menstruation is a common and interesting finding. It may be due to the production of prostaglandins or to the high levels of progesterone present during the secretory phase of the menstrual cycle. Table 3.3 gives important points in the gynaecological history.

Table 3.3 Important points for a gynaecological history

Surgery	Hysterectomy
	Incontinence surgery
	Prolapse repair
	Malignancy ± irradiation
Menstruation	Menopausal status
	Cyclical symptoms?
Current problems	Fibroids
	Prolapse

OBSTETRIC HISTORY

The exact role of pregnancy and parturition in the genesis of urinary symptoms is still unclear. During pregnancy itself, urinary symptoms are very common. Women complain of stress incontinence, frequency, urgency, and voiding difficulties.

During delivery, partial denervation of the pelvic floor musculature and urethral rhabdosphincter may occur, together with damage to the supporting ligaments of the bladder. Reinnervation takes place, however nerve conduction may be prolonged, resulting in muscle weakness. If the correct anatomical position of the bladder neck is lost then this may result in poor pressure transmission to the proximal urethra during episodes of raised intra-abdominal pressure, resulting in incontinence.

It is important to know whether the woman has completed her family, especially if bladder-neck surgery is contemplated. Subsequent pregnancies may result in a recurrence of symptoms and repeat surgery has a higher failure rate than a primary procedure. Table 3.4 gives important points in the obstetric history.

Table 3.4 Important points for an obstetric history

Parity
Mode of delivery, ?trauma
Weight of baby/babies
Symptoms during/after pregnancy
Family complete?

MEDICAL HISTORY

Few medical conditions give rise to incontinence directly, but they may exacerbate existing problems. A systematic enquiry should ensure that important factors are not overlooked. Chronic respiratory disease will exacerbate stress incontinence. Cardiac failure with peripheral oedema may lead to redistribution of fluid at night, causing nocturia and even nocturnal enuresis.

Hypertension is a common condition which itself does not cause urinary incontinence. However, many of the agents used to treat it may affect bladder or urethral function (see below). Chronic constipation may result in frequency, urgency, voiding difficulties, or even overflow incontinence due to pressure effects on the bladder.

A history of rectal soiling together with urinary incontinence suggests a possible neurological cause for both symptoms. The presence of other overt neurological symptoms is uncommon, but when present should be carefully noted and a full neurological assessment carried out by an expert. It is not uncommon for women with multiple sclerosis to present initially to the gynaecologist or urologist with incontinence with or without other neurological deficits. Uncontrolled diabetes mellitus will give rise to urinary frequency due to polyuria, and glycosuria predisposes to urinary tract infection. Long-term diabetes can result in a neuropathic bladder and voiding difficulties.

Table 3.5   Important points for a medical history

Respiratory	COAD/bronchitis
Cardiovascular	Hypertension Heart failure
Gastrointestinal	Constipation Rectal soiling
Neurological	Multiple sclerosis Spinal trauma CVA/neoplasm Disc lesion
Endocrine	Diabetes mellitus
Psychiatric	Mental state Dementia

A brief assessment of the patient's mental state will exclude mental impairment or a major psychiatric disorder. Either might result in inappropriate voiding patterns which may present as 'incontinence'. Table 3.5 gives important points in the medical history.

DRUG HISTORY

Many commonly prescribed drugs used in the treatment of hypertension, anxiety, depression, and psychotic illness will potentially alter detrusor or urethral function. These are summarized in Table 3.6.

Table 3.6 Important points for drug history, noting drugs which alter lower urinary tract function

Drug group	Mechanism	Examples
Diuretics	Increase rate of bladder filling: exacerbate frequency and urgency	Thiazides Frusemide
β-Blockers	Reduce sympathetic supply to detrusor: enhance contractility	Atenolol Propranolol
α-Blockers	Reduce sympathetic supply to urethra: urethral relaxation incontinence	Prazosin
Major tranquillizers	Anticholinergic effect: voiding difficulties	Chlorpromazine
Anxiolytics	Impair urethral function	Benzodiazepines

SOCIAL HISTORY

This is a most important part of the history which is sometimes forgotten in the clinic. The impact of incontinence on a woman's working, family, and sexual life may be dramatic. Embarrassment may result in her becoming virtually housebound, and unable to continue working. Coital incontinence may lead to a fear of intercourse and result in marital problems.

Physical activity is an important determinant of the severity of leakage in women with genuine stress incontinence. A young active woman with mild GSI will complain of more frequent episodes of incontinence than an elderly woman with the same severity of leakage but a more sedentary lifestyle. Many women give up sporting activities because of their urinary incontinence.

DIRECT SYMPTOM QUESTIONNAIRE

It is important that history-taking should be comprehensive and reproducible, so that important information is not overlooked or forgotten. The use of a direct symptom questionnaire will enable data to be collected in a uniform way, which aids diagnosis and facilitates audit and research. An example of such a questionnaire is shown in Fig. 3.1.

PHYSICAL EXAMINATION

An initial general examination may provide useful information for subsequent patient management. The mobility and dexterity of the woman may be limited and result in difficulty in reaching the toilet or removing clothing.

Examination of the cardiorespiratory system is usually unremarkable, however, chronic lung disease and heart failure may be the cause of urinary symptoms. An assessment of the woman's fitness for anaesthesia should be noted. A dementia

URINARY SYMPTOMS DIRECT QUESTIONNAIRE

NAME :   WT :

DATE :

VISIT :

FREQUENCY - DAY times : _____

NOCTURIA   times : _____

(0=NONE   1=OCC   2=OFTEN 3=ALWAYS)

STRESS INCONT :

URGENCY :   _____

URGE INCONT :   _____

WET AT REST :   _____

WET ON STANDING :   _____

WET AT NIGHT :   _____

UNAWARE WETNESS :   _____

PADS / PANTS :   _____

POOR STREAM :   _____

UNABLE STOP FLOW : _____

POST MIC DRIBBLE : _____

STRAIN TO VOID :   _____

INCOMPLETE EMPTY : _____

COUGH :   _____

CONSTIPATION :   _____

RECTAL SOILING :   _____

PAIN MICTURATING : _____

(0=none 1=urethral 2=perineal 3=suprapubic 4=loin)

DYSPAREUNIA : _____

(0=no 1=superficial 2=deep)

Fig. 3.1 An example of a urinary symptom questionnaire.

score may be helpful in the management of elderly incontinent patients.

GYNAECOLOGICAL EXAMINATION

Abdominal and bimanual examination is performed to exclude the presence of a palpable bladder, or an abdomino-pelvic mass which may press on the bladder. Inspection of the vulva will reveal evidence of post-menopausal atrophy, or excoriation due to chronic exposure to urine. A congenital lesion such as epispadias should be recognized on inspection. A profuse vaginal discharge may be the cause of apparent urinary symptoms in some women and may give the impression of urinary leakage.

The sign of stress incontinence may be elicited by asking the woman to cough with a moderately full bladder, preferably while standing. Uterovaginal prolapse and cystocele can be assessed on vaginal examination and Sim's speculum examination in the left lateral position. The presence of a fistula may be difficult to detect clinically and further investigation is mandatory in all suspected cases. The urethra may be palpated along its length for evidence of discharge, tenderness, fibrosis, or a diverticulum. Vaginal mobility should also be assessed as adequate anterior wall elevation is required for certain incontinence operations. The vagina may be narrowed from previous surgery or post-menopausal atrophy.

NEUROLOGICAL EXAMINATION

Ideally a basic neurological examination should be carried out in all women. Tone, power, sensation, and reflexes in the lower limbs should be assessed with particular reference to levels $S_{2,3,4}$. The back is inspected to exclude previous spinal injury or spina bifida occulta.

Special tests to confirm the integrity of sacral reflexes include the bulbocavernosus reflex. The clitoris is gently touched and contraction of the external anal sphincter is produced. Stimulation of the perineum with a pin will yield similar findings. Anal sphincter tone and sensation over the saddle area are simple to assess and provide useful information.

Bonney's test

This test has been used to try to define the cause of incontinence in women with the signs of stress incontinence, and to assess whether surgical intervention is appropriate (Bonney 1923). The forefinger and middle finger of the right hand are inserted into the vagina so as to elevate the vaginal fornices on either side of the bladder neck. The patient is then asked to cough. Absence of urinary leakage during this manoeuvre was thought to indicate that bladder-neck surgery would be effective in alleviating the patient's symptoms. Unfortunately, Bonney's test produces marked compression of the urethra and will prevent leakage of urine in women with or without genuine stress incontinence. It is a useless test and should be avoided.

The 'Q-tip' test

A moistened cotton bud or 'Q-tip' is inserted into the urethra. The patient is asked to strain and the change in angle of the Q-tip is measured. The change in angle is proportional to the degree of bladder-neck descent on the Valsalva manoeuvre (Crystle *et al.* 1971). Although this anatomical defect is associated with genuine stress incontinence it is not diagnostic, and may occur in women with uterovaginal prolapse without urinary incontinence. This test is used commonly in North America but is not considered to be clinically useful in the United Kingdom.

REFERENCES

Bonney, V. (1923). On diurnal incontinence of urine in women. *J. Obstet Gynaecol. Br. Emp.*, **30**, 358.

Crystle, C.D., Charme, L.S., and Copeland, W.E. (1971). Q-tip test in stress urinary incontinence. *Obstet. Gynecol.*, **38**, 313.

4

Investigation of lower urinary tract dysfunction

INTRODUCTION

The investigations of lower urinary tract dysfunction range from simple procedures performed in the GP surgery to sophisticated investigations only available in tertiary referral centres. Each

Table 4.1 Investigations for lower urinary tract dysfunction

Non-specialist investigations

Mid-stream specimen of urine
Frequency–volume chart
Pad test

Specialist investigations

Uroflowmetry
Cystometry
Videocystourethrography
Ambulatory urodynamics
Urethral pressure profilometry
Urethral electrical conductance
Electromyography
Micturating cystography
Intravenous urography
Ultrasonography
Cystourethroscopy

---

investigation has its own appropriate place in the assessment of lower urinary tract dysfunction, and assessment techniques should be tailored to the individual patient's needs. The various tests which are available are shown in Table 4.1.

MID-STREAM SPECIMEN OF URINE

Urinary tract infections are not a common cause of incontinence but they will certainly aggravate any symptoms which are present. In addition, the presence of a urinary tract infection may invalidate the results of any investigations performed, and therefore the presence of urinary tract infection should always be checked for prior to investigation. A nitrate-stick test can be used as a screening test for urinary tract infection but the diagnosis is made from a clean, mid-stream specimen of urine in which a pure growth of greater than 10^5 organisms per ml of urine is taken to signify an infection (Kass 1957).

FREQUENCY–VOLUME CHARTS

Frequency–volume charts can be used to assess voiding patterns objectively. They are also useful in determining fluid intake and urine output and for documenting urinary incontinence and periods of urgency (Abrams *et al*. 1990). There are no recommendations as to the length of time they should span.

Several different types have been described with recordings from two days up to seven days. We use a five-day chart (Fig. 4.1). From a frequency–volume chart, an increased number of voids due to excessive fluid intake or diuretic therapy, or increased night voiding due to drinking late at night, can easily be assessed. The severity of incontinence can be determined by the number of wet episodes recorded. Frequency-volume charts are also useful in teaching bladder drill and to monitor the effects of treatment.

FREQUENCY VOLUME CHART

NAME :
DATE :
VISIT :

Time	Day 1			Day 2			Day 3			Day 4			Day 5		
	IN	OUT	W	IN	OUT	W	IN	OUT	W	IN	OUT	W	IN	OUT	W
6am															
7am															
8am															
9am															
10am															
11am															
12															
1pm															
2pm															
3pm															
4pm															
5pm															
6pm															
7pm															
8pm															
9pm															
10pm															
11pm															
12															
1am															
2am															
3am															
4am															
5am															

Fig. 4.1 An example of a frequency–volume chart.

PAD TESTS

Pad tests were first described by Sutherst *et al.* (1981). They are used to verify incontinence and to quantify the degree of urine loss. The standard pad test, as recommended by the International Continence Society, involves placing a pre-weighed pad in the underwear. With this pad in place a series of manoeuvres are carried out over a one-hour period and the pad is then re-weighed (Abrams *et al.* 1990). A weight gain of greater than one gram signifies incontinence. It is recommended that the subject takes a fluid load of 500 ml prior to the test. There are many variations, however, with some investigators using different test times and others instilling a standard volume into the bladder prior to commencing the test.

Recently it has been suggested that 24 hour and 48 hour home pad tests are more representative. In these, the woman carries out her normal daily activities while wearing a pre-weighed pad. Each pad is weighed and the total amount of leakage in a 24- or 48-hour period can be assessed.

URODYNAMIC INVESTIGATIONS

Urodynamic investigations assess function rather than structure of the lower urinary tract. They comprise a group of tests with which all other methods of investigation must be compared. This is the method by which diagnoses are made and, indeed, the classification of lower urinary tract disorders is based on urodynamic parameters. Although symptoms will cause the patients to present and simple objective tests will define abnormalities in voiding patterns or the presence of incontinence, they will not determine the underlying pathophysiology.

Several authors have demonstrated in prospective studies that symptoms do not accurately reflect lower urinary tract dysfunction. Jarvis *et al.* (1980) compared clinical diagnosis with the urodynamic diagnosis in 100 women. The referring gynaecologist made a diagnosis of genuine stress incontinence in 41

women and detrusor instability in 59 women on symptoms
alone. On urodynamic investigation, 41 women had a diagnosis
of genuine stress incontinence, 35 had detrusor instability, 7 had
mixed stress incontinence and detrusor instability, and 17 had
sensory urgency. There was agreement in 28 cases (68 per cent)
of genuine stress incontinence and 30 cases (51 per cent) of
detrusor instability.

Figure 4.2 shows the prevalence of urinary symptoms for
those women with a urodynamic diagnosis of genuine stress
incontinence ($n = 41$) and detrusor instability ($n = 35$). Indeed,
although nearly all the women with genuine stress incontinence
complained of stress incontinence, 46 per cent of them also
complained of urgency. Of the 35 women with detrusor instability, 26 per cent complained of stress incontinence.

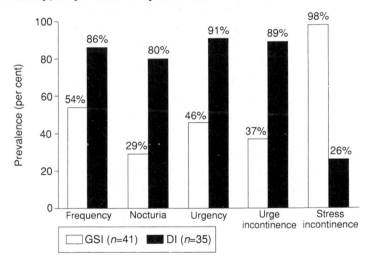

Fig. 4.2 The prevalence of urinary symptoms for women with genuine
stress incontinence (GSI) and those with detrusor instability (DI).

Conversely, it has been shown that where stress incontinence
is the sole symptom, then genuine stress incontinence is likely to
be present in over 90 per cent of women. However, patients
rarely present with solitary symptoms.

UROFLOWMETRY

Uroflowmetry is an essential part of any urodynamic assessment. It is relatively simple and is non-invasive. The first flow meter was described by von Garrelts (1956). The original design utilized a strain-gauge-weighing transducer placed under a cylindrical receptacle into which the patient voids. The weight of fluid is electronically converted to give a simultaneous flow rate. In addition the total volume of fluid can be measured. It is important to appreciate that the strain gauge is in fact measuring a change in mass and for this reason it needs to be calibrated for

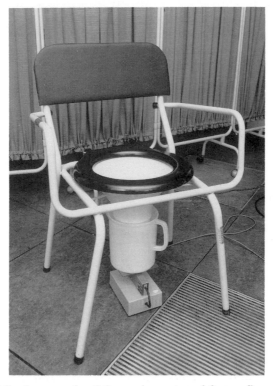

Fig. 4.3   An example of the equipment used for uroflowmetry.

fluid of the correct density. Other commonly used devices include an electronic dip stick, a rotating disc, ultrasound, and the displacement of air from a container. Figure 4.3 shows the commode seat and flowmeter used in our unit, which is of the weighing transducer type.

To obtain a record of flow parameters, the patient is asked to void into the flowmeter once her bladder is comfortably full. Preferably this should be carried out in private. The maximum flow rate and the volume voided are recorded. In addition the average flow rate, the flow time, and the time to maximum flow may be determined (Fig. 4.4).

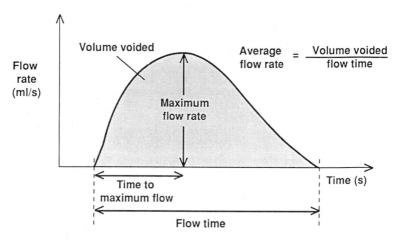

Fig. 4.4 Information obtained from uroflowmetry.

The normal trace is bell shaped with a peak flow of at least 15 ml/s for a volume of at least 150 ml of urine. A normal trace is shown in Fig. 4.5. A reduced maximum flow rate may be merely due to an inadequate voided volume or voiding difficulties (Fig. 4.6). Voiding difficulties due to a hypotonic detrusor or outflow obstruction cannot be differentiated by uroflowmetry alone. In addition the shape of the curve may be altered and may suggest evidence of abdominal straining on voiding. It is very important to record the volume voided as small volumes will

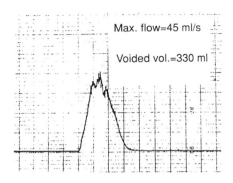

Fig. 4.5 A normal flow-rate curve.

lead to low peak flow rates. Haylen *et al.* (1989) have produced nomograms for the peak flow rate and average flow rate in normal men and women, taking the volume voided into account.

Further analysis of flow rates involves pressure flow studies and these will be discussed in combination with cystometry.

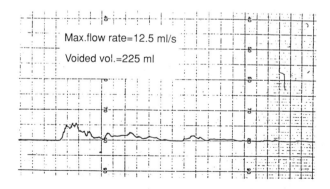

Fig. 4.6 A flow-rate curve demonstrating a decreased maximum flow rate and a prolonged flow time.

CYSTOMETRY

Cystometry is the measurement of the pressure/volume relation-ship of the bladder. The first cystometer was described by Mosso and Pellacani in 1882. A water manometer was used to measure the intravesical pressure at increasing bladder volumes. The pressure was recorded on a smoked drum. This form of cyst-ometry is known as single-channel or simple cystometry.

In simple cystometry the intravesical (total bladder) pressure is measured while the bladder is filled (Fig. 4.7). It is not entirely accurate as it assumes that the detrusor pressure approximates the intravesical pressure. However, as the bladder is an intra-

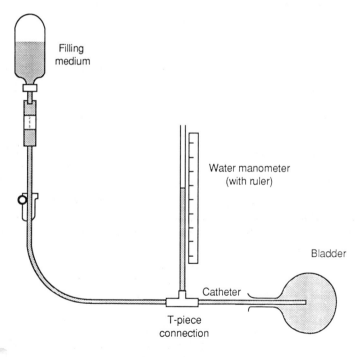

Fig. 4.7 Diagrammatic representation of simple cystometry.

abdominal organ, the detrusor is subject to changes in intra-abdominal pressure which may lead to inaccurate diagnoses. Subtracted cystometry involves measurement of both the intra-vesical and intra-abdominal pressure simultaneously. Electronic subtraction of the latter from the former enables the detrusor pressure to be determined.

Subtracted provocative cystometry

A filling catheter (12 French Jacques) and a pressure-measuring catheter (1 mm plastic tube) are passed into the bladder and a pressure balloon on a 2 mm fluid tube is inserted into the rectum. The urinary residual is measured. The bladder is normally filled with the patient in the supine or sitting position and the first sensation of desire to void and bladder capacity are recorded. The woman then stands up and the filling catheter is removed. In the erect position she is asked to cough and also to heel bounce, and any rise in detrusor pressure or leakage is noted. She is then asked to pass urine and the detrusor pressure is measured. During voiding she is told to suddenly interrupt her stream. The urethral sphincter and pelvic floor, which are under somatic innervation, will contract immediately but the smooth muscle of the detrusor will continue to contract for a short period of time. The resulting contraction is known as the iso-metric detrusor contraction. At the end of the investigation the patient is asked to empty her bladder completely and the residual volume is measured. Figure 4.8(a) and (b) show equipment used for subtracted cystometry. Figure 4.9 is a diagrammatic repres-entation of subtracted cystometry and Fig. 4.10 shows the trace of a normal cystometrogram.

The normal values for subtracted cystometry have been docu-mented. A residual volume of greater than 50 ml is considered to be abnormal and persistently large urinary residuals are a sign of voiding difficulties.

The normal first sensation occurs when the bladder contains between 150 and 250 ml and the normal bladder capacity is 400 to 600 ml. During filling to 500 ml, the detrusor pressure does not normally rise by more than 15 cm H_2O. A rise greater than this indicates low compliance (Fig. 4.11). Detrusor instability is indicated by detrusor contractions causing a rise in detrusor pressure usually greater than 15 cm H_2O, associated with symptoms, when the individual is trying to inhibit micturition. If these rises in pressure occur on filling they are termed systolic contractions (Fig. 4.12) and if on provocation, provoked detrusor contractions (Fig. 4.11). However, due to the fact that filling via a catheter may be considered provocative in itself, the term 'phasic detrusor contraction' is often used to encompass both terms.

Leakage occurs if the detrusor pressure exceeds the urethral pressure. If there is no pressure rise on filling and the patient leaks because of raised intra-abdominal pressure without a rise in detrusor pressure, then a diagnosis of genuine stress incontinence/urethral sphincter incompetence is made.

Various abnormalities can be diagnosed from the voiding phase of the cystometrogram. A low voiding pressure with a reduced flow rate suggests a diagnosis of voiding difficulty due

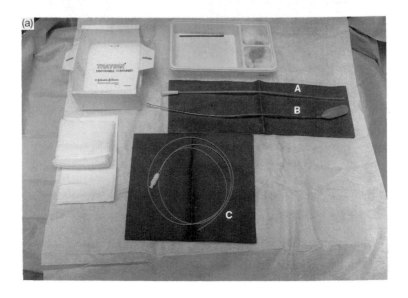

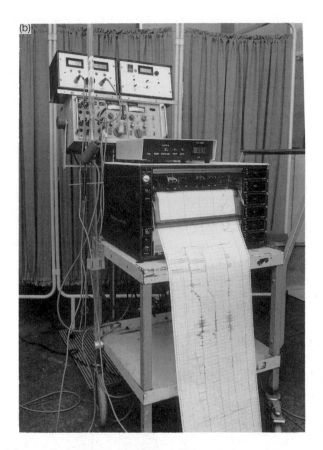

Fig. 4.8 (a) Catheters required for subtracted cystometry: A, Size 12 French filling catheter; B, Rectal pressure line (balloon catheter); C, Intravesical pressure line. (b) Urodynamic equipment.

to detrusor hypotonia. A raised voiding pressure with a reduced flow rate suggests a diagnosis of voiding difficulty due to outflow obstruction. However, in the case of outflow obstruction, the detrusor will, with time, often decompensate such that it becomes hypotonic, and may present with a low flow rate and low voiding pressure.

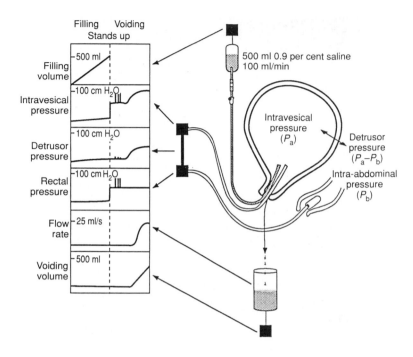

Fig. 4.9 Diagrammatic representation of subtracted cystometry.

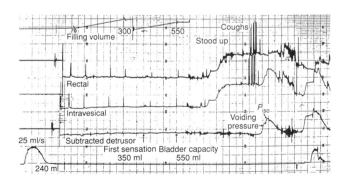

Fig. 4.10 A normal cystometrogram.

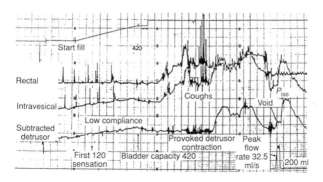

Fig. 4.11 A cystometrogram demonstrating low compliance and provoked detrusor contraction.

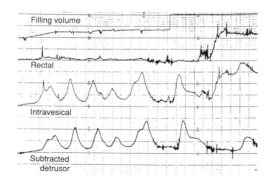

Fig. 4.12 A cystometrogram demonstrating systolic detrusor contractions.

A cystometrogram is necessary to make a diagnosis of detrusor instability as it is a urodynamic diagnosis. Genuine stress incontinence may be diagnosed by exclusion. Cystometry is particularly useful in differentiating between cough-induced detrusor instability and genuine stress incontinence.

METHODS OF TESTING

Several studies have compared single-channel and subtracted cystometry. The conclusion of most of these studies was that single-channel cystometry may be used as a screening test but would appear to over-diagnose detrusor instability. Various factors will affect the results of cystometric investigations: the method of pressure measurement, the filling medium, the rate of filling, and whether it was incremental or continuous. In addition, repeated tests may affect results.

Pressure transducers

Different types of pressure-measuring devices have been described. The water manometer originally used does not facilitate a continuous pressure reading but provides incremental pressure measurements during filling.

Two types of pressure transducer are used nowadays: fluid-filled catheters attached to an external pressure transducer and solid-state microtip pressure tranducers mounted on a catheter. The fluid-filled catheters can have a balloon mounted on the end to prevent blockage when they are used to measure intra-rectal or intra-vaginal pressure. The advantages of fluid-filled pressure catheters are that they are less expensive and more durable. The advantage of microtip pressure transducers is that they have a faster response time. The expense and lack of durability of these catheters are a distinct disadvantage.

Pressure recordings are made either on a paper chart recorder or on to computer software.

Filling medium

The filling medium can be either gas or liquid. Originally water was used but nowadays 0.9 per cent saline is the most commonly used filling medium. If simultaneous radiological screening is to be carried out, then a radio-opaque filling medium such as

Urografin can be used. Gas cystometry is popular in North America. Air was the original gas used but has now been largely replaced by carbon dioxide.

The advantage of gas cystometry is that it is quick, clean, and easy to perform. However, it has many disadvantages: it is only possible to carry out single-channel cystometry and most authors have found it to have poor reproducibility, giving more diagnoses of detrusor instability than liquid cystometry. The apparently higher incidence of detrusor instability may be due to the fact that carbon dioxide dissolves in urine to form carbonic acid which is an irritant to the bladder. In addition, gas cystometry will only allow assessment of the bladder during filling as voiding studies are not possible.

Mode of filling

Other factors which may affect results are the rate of filling, the temperature of the fluid, and whether filling is incremental or continuous.

The temperature of the fluid has no effect on results as long as it lies between room temperature and body temperature. However, a cold filling medium will result in an increased incidence of detrusor instability. This is the basis of the Bors ice-cold water test.

It has been repeatedly shown that cystometry performed in different positions will lead to differing rates of detection of detrusor instability—filling in a standing or sitting position will result in a higher incidence than filling in the supine position.

Finally it is important to realize that cystometry gives poor reproducibility with regard to detrusor instability as the patient may exhibit abnormalities on one occasion which are not present on another occasion. It is therefore important to look at the results of investigations in the context of the patients symptomatology and if necessary repeat investigations when the results are unexpectedly normal.

Video-cystourethrography (VCU)

If Urografin is used to fill the bladder, then the lower urinary tract can be visualized during cystometry using X-ray screening usually with an image intensifier. After filling the bladder, the patient is stood erect on an X-ray screening table. She is asked to cough with a full bladder, so that both the extent of bladder-base descent and leakage of contrast medium can be evaluated (Fig. 4.13). During voiding, bladder morphology can be assessed —vesico-ureteric reflex, trabeculation, and diverticulae (Fig. 4.14) should be noted. Rarely, a urethral diverticulum or a vesico-vaginal fistula may be identified. VCU is a sophisticated mode of investigation first described by Bates *et al.* (1970) and prob-

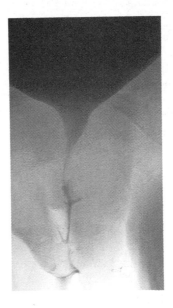

Fig. 4.13 A videocystourethrogram demonstrating bladder-neck opening and urinary leakage on coughing (this patient had a diagnosis of genuine stress incontinence).

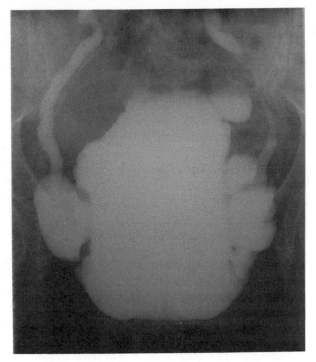

Fig. 4.14 A videocystourethrogram demonstrating bladder diverticula, trabeculation, and bilateral ureteric reflux.

ably currently the 'Gold standard' for the investigation of lower urinary tract function (Turner-Warwick 1979).

However, it is an expensive technique as it requires access to radiology department and considerable expertise. For these reasons many centres perform subtracted provocative cystometry without the addition of X-ray screening.

Ambulatory urodynamics

Recently it has been suggested that the poor correlation between symptoms and urodynamic findings is due to the mode of investigation, with subtracted cystometry being too insensitive in the detection of detrusor instability. Ambulatory urodynamics enables bladder function to be recorded over a longer period of time than conventional urodynamics.

Different techniques have been described, either involving measurement of the intravesical and urethral pressures or, in addition to these, measuring the rectal pressure. Recordings can be made on a 24 h tape which is reviewed subsequently. Workers in this field have suggested that ambulatory urodynamics is more physiological as the assessment takes place during normal daily activities and is more sensitive in the detection of detrusor instability. However, as yet it is not a routine test in the assessment of lower urinary tract function.

Urethral pressure profilometry

The first report of urethral pressure measurements was by Bonney (1923) by a technique known as retrograde sphincterometry. The advent of solid-state microtransducers enabled more accurate pressure measurements to be obtained. A catheter with two microtip pressure transducers a set distance apart is gradually withdrawn at a constant rate along the urethra, enabling simultaneous recording of the intravesical and intraurethral pressures (Fig. 4.15).

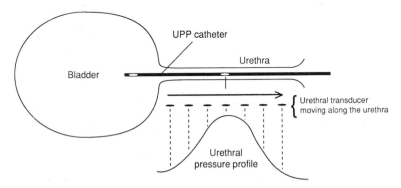

Fig. 4.15 Diagrammatic representation of urethral pressure profilometry (UPP).

Electronic subtraction of these recordings can be made. Many different parameters of the resultant trace can be analysed. It is important to appreciate that the technique is a measure of urethral function and not detrusor function as only the intra-vesical pressure is recorded.

The profile can be assessed both at rest and during stress. During rest, the standard parameters analysed include the maximum urethral pressure (MUP), the maximum urethral closure pressure (MUCP), functional urethral length (FUL), and anatomical urethral length (UL).

The catheter can then be withdrawn at a standard rate while the patient gives repeated coughs thus producing a stress–pressure profile. The same measurements can then be recorded. In addition a loss of urethral closure pressure on raised intra-abdominal

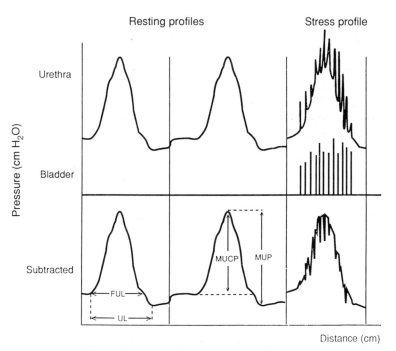

Fig. 4.16 A urethral pressure profile trace.

pressure can be noted (Hilton and Stanton 1983). A normal urethral pressure profile trace is shown in Fig. 4.16.

The use of urethral pressure profile profilometry in the diagnosis of lower urinary tract dysfunction is controversial. The resting profile cannot be used to diagnose genuine stress incontinence. Although the maximum urethral pressure and maximum urethral closure pressure are significantly reduced in women with GSI compared with normal controls, there is considerable overlap between groups. A negative stress pressure profile is said to occur when the intravesical pressure exceeds the intra-urethral pressure with a cough. However, it has been shown that the size of the cough influences the stress curve, thus making its analysis unreliable.

Urethral pressure profilometry can also be used in women with voiding difficulties. The upper limit of 'normal' is uncertain and falls with increasing age, but a markedly raised maximum urethral closure pressure in association with a low peak flow rate would indicate outflow obstruction.

Thus it would appear that urethral pressure profilometry is a useful tool in the investigation of lower urinary tract dysfunction. However, to date normal ranges have not been well documented.

Urethral electrical conductance

In urethral electrical conductance (UEC) tests, a 7 French flexible probe with two ring electrodes separated by 1 mm is positioned within the urethra. It measures movement of urine along the urethra by registering a change in the conductivity reading. As the catheter is withdrawn a profile is obtained. This can be used to measure bladder-neck activity and urethral closure mechanisms (Plevnik *et al.* 1983).

In distal urethral electrical conductance, the electrodes are placed 1.5 cm from the external urethral meatus. Different patterns of conductivity are associated with different urodynamic diagnoses. It has been recommended as a screening test for incontinence. This technique has not as yet gained widespread popularity.

Electromyography

This can be used to look at the integrity of a muscle and its nerve supply. Electrical impulses in muscle fibres are measured during spontaneous activity or following neural stimulation. Two main varieties are used in the investigation of lower urinary tract dysfunction. In surface EMG, the pudendal nerve is stimulated and potentials measured on the skin overlying a group of muscle fibres. It is inaccurate as potentials measured in the levator ani do not necessarily represent abnormalities in the rhabdosphincter urethrae. Single-fibre EMG involves recording of individual muscle fibres of the rhabdosphincter and the nerve latency is measured. It is used to look at denervation of motor units. Genuine stress incontinence may be due to partial denervation of the pelvic floor musculature and rhabdosphincter and is characterized by increased motor latencies (Smith *et al.* 1989). EMG is most useful when a neurological abnormality is suspected.

Imaging of the lower urinary tract

The lower urinary tract can be visualized with X-rays, ultrasound, via a cystoscope, and, most recently, with magnetic resonance imaging. X-ray screening as part of the urodynamic investigation enhances dynamic assessment of the lower urinary tract. Combined with cystometry it is known as videocysto-urethrography.

Micturition cystography

This will give similar morphological information to that obtained when X-ray screening is used as part of the urodynamic investigation. However, it is more useful to record anatomical abnormalities in association with changes in detrusor pressures, thus the combined investigation (VCU) is usually preferable. Micturition cystography may be useful in the diagnosis of fistulae or to diagnose a urethral diverticulum.

Intravenous urography (IVU)

An IVU (Fig. 4.17) is employed in cases of haematuria, recurrent urinary tract infections, outflow obstruction, known voiding difficulties, or vesico-ureteric reflux. In addition, ureteric fistulae and filling defects in association with pathology such as a transitional-cell carcinoma or stones may be seen. It is specifically used for looking at the upper urinary tract, and in many centres nowadays has been superseded by ultrasound.

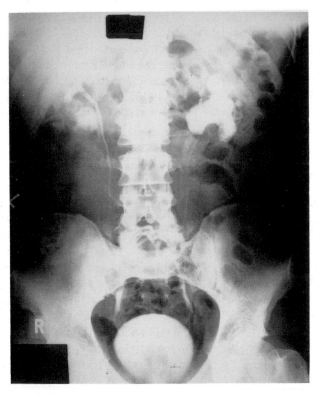

Fig. 4.17 An intravenous urogram demonstrating bilateral duplex collecting systems and a large left-sided staghorn calculus.

Ultrasound

Ultrasound is a non-invasive technique. Both abdominal and vaginal ultrasound are routinely used for determining bladder volumes (Figs 4.18 and 4.19). The bladder capacity and urinary residual can be estimated. Ultrasound is also used to assess the upper tracts, when looking for ureteric dilatation and renal tumours. Its role in examining the lower urinary tract in the diagnosis of urinary incontinence has not been established. The use of vaginal ultrasonography to differentiate GSI from detrusor instability has been suggested by several authors but is not widely accepted (Quinn 1990). It is important to appreciate that although ultrasound examination enables us to look at the anatomy and detect morphological abnormalities of the lower urinary tract, it cannot replace those investigations which assess dynamic pressure changes of the lower urinary tract. In addition, the ultrasound image is really not as clear as that produced by radiological screening.

Cysto-urethroscopy

This is normally carried out under general anaesthesia but if a flexible cystoscope is used then local anaesthesia can be used. It should be performed where there is a history of haematuria, recurrent urinary tract infections, sensory urgency, or marked urinary symptoms of frequency, urgency, or dysuria with normal urodynamic investigations.

A papilloma or bladder stone may be seen. Inflamed mucosa suggests chronic infection. Shallow ulcers may be due to interstitial cystitis and pale mucosa is seen when atrophic trigonitis has occurred after the menopause. In addition, biopsies can be taken at the time of the investigation. A biopsy will enable transitional-cell carcinoma to be diagnosed. Histology may also reveal chronic inflammation or numerous mast cells typical of interstitial cystitis.

Magnetic resonance imaging

This is a relatively new tool and its role in assessing the anatomy of the lower urinary tract is still in the experimental stages (Klutke *et al.* 1990). The fine detail that it reveals may be useful in determining damage to the urethral sphincter mechanisms in cases of genuine stress incontinence.

SUMMARY

There are many investigations of lower urinary tract dysfunction but subtracted cystometry remains the most useful in making an

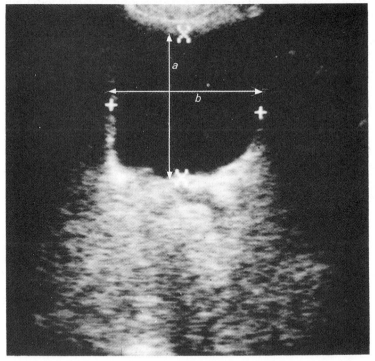

Fig. 4.18   Transverse abdominal ultrasound scan of a urinary residual. Bladder volume $= a \times b \times c \times 0.7$, where c is obtained from Fig. 4.19.

accurate diagnosis. Other tests, however, make useful contributions in understanding the underlying pathology which has lead to lower urinary tract dysfunction. The different tests and their established indications are outlined in Table 4.2. A summary of urodynamic criteria used to make a diagnosis is shown in Table 4.3.

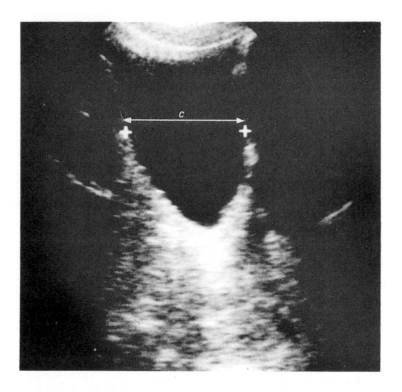

Fig. 4.19 Longitudinal abdominal ultrasound scan of a urinary residual. Bladder volume $= a \times b \times c \times 0.7$, where a and b are obtained from Fig. 4.18.

Table 4.2 Investigations leading to a diagnosis

	Frequency	Incontinence	Stress incontinence	Urgency/ urge incontinence	Voiding difficulty	Fistulae
MSSU	*	*		*	*	
Freq./Vol.	*			*		
Flow rate					*	
Cystometry	*	*	*	*	*	
VCU	*	*	*	*	*	*
UPP			(*)		*	
EMG			(*)		*	
USS	*				*	

Table 4.3   Making a urodynamic diagnosis

Parameter	Pathophysiology
Reduced peak flow rate (normal > 15 ml/s)	Inadequate volume passed Detrusor hypotonia (associated with low voiding pressure) Urethral obstruction (high voiding pressure)
First sensation (normal 150–250 ml) and bladder capacity (normal 400–600 ml)	*Decreased* Sensory urgency (if no abnormal rise in detrusor pressure) Detrusor instability *Increased* Associated with overflow incontinence
Rise in detrusor pressure of > 15 cm H_2O	Gradual rise on filling: low compliance Peaked rise on filling: systolic DI Rise on coughing: provoked DI
Leakage	Without a rise in pressure: GSI With a rise in pressure: DI Fistula
Urethral pressure profile parameters	Raised: Outflow obstruction Lowered: Suggest GSI

REFERENCES

Abrams, P., Blaivas, J.G., Stanton, S.L., and Andersen, J.T. (1990). The standardisation of terminology of lower urinary tract function. *Br. J. Obstet. Gynaecol.* (Suppl.) **6**, 1–16.

Bates, C.P., Whiteside, C.G., and Turner-Warwick, R. (1970). Synchronous cine/pressure/flow cystourethrography with special reference to stress and urge incontinence. *Br. J. Urol.*, **42**, 714–23.

Bonney, V. (1923). On diurnal incontinence of urine in women. *J. Obstet. Gynaecol. Br. Emp.*, **30**, 358–65.

Haylen, B.T., Ashby, D., Sutherst, J.R., Frazer, M.I., and West, C.R. (1989). Maximum and average flow rates in normal male and female populations—the Liverpool nomogans. *Br. J. Urol.*, **64**, 30–8.

Hilton, P. and Stanton, S.L. (1983). Urethral pressure measurement by microtransducer: the results in symptom-free women and in those with genuine stress incontinence. *Br. J. Obstet. Gynaecol.*, **90**, 919–33.

Jarvis, G.J., Hall, S., Stamp, S., Miller, D.R., and Johnson, A. (1980). An assessment of urodynamic examination in incontinent women. *Br. J. Obstet. Gynaecol.*, **87**, 893–6.

Kass, E.H. (1957). Bacteriuria and the diagnosis of infections of the urinary tract. *A.M.A. Archives Int. Med.*, **100**, 709–14.

Klutke, C., Golomb, J., Barbaric, Z., and Raz, S. (1990). The anatomy of stress incontinence: magnetic resonance imaging of the female bladder neck and urethra. *J. Urol.*, **143**, 563–6.

Plevnik, S., Vrtacnik, P., and Janez, P. (1983). Detection of fluid entry into the urethra by electrical impedence measurement: electric fluid bridge test. *Clin. Phys. Physiol. Meas.*, **4**, 309–13.

Quinn, M.J. (1990). Vaginal ultrasound and urinary stress incontinence. *Contemp. Rev. Obstet. Gynaecol.*, **2**, 104–10.

Smith, A.R.B., Hosker, G.L., and Warrell, D.W. (1989). The role of partial denervation of the pelvic floor in the aetiology of genito-urinary prolapse and stress incontinence of urine. A neurophysiological study. *Br. J. Obstet. Gynaecol.*, **96**, 24–8.

Sutherst, J.L., Brown, M., and Shawer, M. (1981). Assessing the severity of urine incontinence in women by weighing perineal pads. *Lancet*, **i**, 1128–30.

Turner-Warwick, R. (1979). The evaluation of urodynamic function. *Urol. Clin. N. Am.1*, **6**, 51–4.

von Garrelts, B. (1956). Analysis of micturition: a new method of recording the voiding of the bladder. *Acta Chirurgica Scand.*, **112**, 326–40.

5

Who to investigate and how

INTRODUCTION

We have outlined all the investigations available in making an accurate diagnosis of the pathophysiology of lower urinary tract dysfunction. Not all women, however, will require extensive investigation prior to treatment.

STRESS INCONTINENCE

If the symptoms are suggestive of genuine stress incontinence then those women not wanting surgery can have a trial of conservative treatment prior to investigation. Pelvic floor exercises should be taught and possibly combined with hormone replacement therapy in post-menopausal women. If there is not considerable improvement in the symptoms then subtracted cystometry should be performed. Although conservative treatment will not be detrimental, it is time consuming for a patient to perform pelvic floor exercises and in addition it is discouraging to have ineffective treatment for any length of time.

If the woman complains of the sole symptom of stress incontinence without any irritative bladder symptoms, then there is over a 90 per cent chance that she has genuine stress incontinence. However, it is unwise to operate without at least excluding voiding difficulties as results may be disastrous. A peak flow rate and estimation of post-micturition urinary residual are the minimum investigations required prior to surgery.

In most women with stress incontinence, subtracted cystometry without fluoroscopy is adequate. However, in cases of failed surgery, videocystourethroscopy is the investigation of choice as the morphology of the bladder and urethra and the amount of descent of the bladder neck should be visualized to plan the appropriate operation.

Finally it is important to remember that stress incontinence may be the presenting symptom in overflow incontinence and failure to treat this condition in the short term may result not only in renal damage but also jeopardize possible recovery of a hypotonic detrusor.

IRRITATIVE BLADDER SYMPTOMS

If the main symptoms are of frequency and urgency with or without dysuria then it may be reasonable to assume that the underlying condition is detrusor instability or sensory urgency and to treat accordingly. However, although hormone replacement therapy is unlikely to have any lower urinary tract side effects, drugs with anticholinergic side effects will compromise detrusor function and may lead to the development of voiding difficulties.

Initial simple investigations include an assessment of fluid intake and a mid-stream specimen of urine in all cases. The urinary residual should be checked to exclude voiding difficulties, preferably combined with uroflowmetry. The woman can then be treated with anticholinergic agents and if there is symptomatic improvement, further investigations will not be required. To be effective, anticholinergic agents must be given in doses which will give rise to unpleasant side effects, and therefore inappropriate treatment for any length of time is not recommended.

In most cases subtracted cystometry is sufficient but if a neurological cause is suspected or the detrusor contractions are of large magnitude, then videocystourethroscopy is the investigation of choice to look for vesico-ureteric reflux and bladder trabeculation.

III

Treatment

If a diagnosis of sensory urgency is made on cystometry but there is poor response to initial treatment, a cystoscopy and bladder-base biopsy should be carried out to exclude interstitial cystitis. A cystoscopy is mandatory in all cases presenting with haematuria.

VOIDING DIFFICULTIES

When there are symptoms of voiding difficulties with or without other lower urinary tract symptoms, complete investigation is necessary. The diagnosis will be confirmed with uroflowmetry and estimation of urinary residual, and the different causes will be differentiated by subtracted cystometry. Visualization of the lower urinary tract will be of benefit to look for ureteric dilatation and the morphology of the urethra. The need for urethral pressure profilometry is controversial but we would recommend it to confirm urethral obstruction and so avoid unnecessary urethral dilatations.

SUMMARY

In summary, intensive investigation is not required in all cases but treatment without knowing the underlying pathology can result in a despondent patient. In all conditions certain basic investigations, such as sending a mid-stream specimen of urine for culture, should be performed prior to treatment. Finally, as the majority of women will present with mixed symptoms, treatment without investigation is unsatisfactory and will often be inappropriate.

6

Treatment of genuine stress incontinence

INTRODUCTION

Genuine stress incontinence and detrusor instability are the commonest causes of urinary incontinence in women. As the appropriate treatment of these two conditions is completely different it is of paramount importance that an accurate diagnosis is made before therapy is instituted. This is particularly relevant when surgery is contemplated, as the results may be irreversible. As genuine stress incontinence and detrusor instability are both very common it is not unusual for them to coexist and this presents a management problem. In this section we will be outlining the treatment of genuine stress incontinence. This is primarily surgical but conservative treatment may be appropriate in some cases.

CONSERVATIVE TREATMENT

Conservative treatment is reserved for those cases which are unsuitable for surgery. In the younger woman who has not completed her family, conservative therapy is used because a further pregnancy may result in a recurrence of the condition and multiple operations are often unsuccessful. It is also used in cases of mild genuine stress incontinence but is unlikely to be curative in more severe cases where surgical correction of the anatomical defect is necessary. Occasionally the anaesthetic risk to a patient will be too great for surgery to be safely undertaken but with modern anaesthetics and good post-operative care, this is rare. In addition where the anaesthetic risk is too great, epidural analgesia will be sufficient in many cases.

Conservative treatment (Table 6.1) usually involves some kind of physiotherapy with or without electrical devices. There are

Table 6.1   Conservative treatment of genuine stress incontinence

---

Kegel exercises
Cones
Electrical treatment: Faradism
                                      Interferential therapy
Perineometer
Hormone replacement therapy: Oestrogens
α-Sympathomimetics: Phenylpropanolamine

---

many varieties of pelvic floor exercise. The traditional type are Kegel exercises which involve contraction of the pelvic floor five times per hour, every hour of the day (Kegel 1949). They are traditionally taught postnatally to improve the strength of the pelvic floor after delivery. Ideally they should be taught on a one-to-one basis and a vaginal examination should be carried out to confirm that the woman is indeed contracting the correct muscles.

More recently, vaginal cones have been evaluated (Peattie *et al.* 1988) (Fig. 6.1). These are graded weights which are inserted into the vagina for 15 minutes at the beginning and the end of each day. Pelvic floor contraction is essential to keep the weights in the vagina as contracting the abdominal or gluteal muscles will not aid retention of the cones. By gradually increasing the weights, the strength of the pelvic floor contractions will increase.

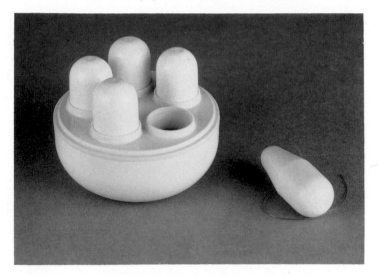

Fig. 6.1 A set of vaginal cones.

Electrical stimulation can take the form of faradism or interferential therapy. Faradism is a technique in which a vaginal
plug is used to apply a direct current to the pelvic floor. In interferential therapy two high frequency voltages are directed
towards the pelvic floor from opposing directions and at the
point of cross-over there will be a low-frequency effect causing
pelvic floor contraction (Laycock 1988). Both techniques work
via two mechanisms—by causing pelvic floor contractions the
strength of the pelvic floor will be increased and, in addition,
they will help to teach the woman which muscle groups to contract during pelvic floor exercises.

In all types of physiotherapy it is necessary to assess improvement in pelvic floor contractions. This can be done either on
digital vaginal examination or with the use of a perineometer
(Shepherd and Montgomery 1983). The perineometer (Fig. 6.2)
is placed in the vagina and an objective recording of pelvic floor
muscle strength is made. The perineometer can also be used to
aid pelvic floor exercises by enabling the woman to gauge the
strength of the contraction which she generates.

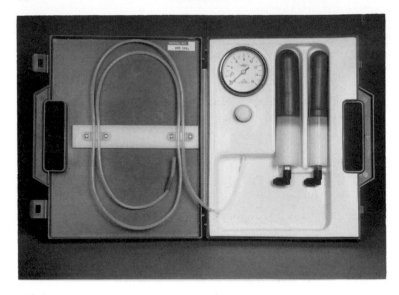

Fig. 6.2 A perineometer.

Simple measures can be instituted to improve genuine stress incontinence. Any precipitating or aggravating factors should be reduced as far as possible. Although increased body weight does not cause genuine stress incontinence, a reduction in weight may lessen the amount of leakage. Any chronic cough should be treated as this will compound the problem. Some women with mild genuine stress incontinence derive benefit from the use of a sanitary tampon or sponge during periods of marked exertion (e.g. sporting activities). A ring pessary may be useful in the elderly as it will result in some elevation of the bladder neck.

Oestrogen can be used in post-menopausal women although it is of no proven benefit in genuine stress incontinence (Cardozo 1990). Oestrogen does improve the strength of collagen fibres and so should improve the supporting ligaments of the bladder neck and the strength of pelvic floor contractions. In addition, epithelial surfaces which are better oestrogenized and more vascular should facilitate urethral closure by forming a watertight seal. Oestrogen therapy is normally used in conjunction with other forms of treatment. The smooth muscle of the bladder neck has α-adrenergic innervation which results in contraction. Drugs such as phenylpropanolamine have been tried but tend to be of little benefit as the sole treatment in cases of genuine stress incontinence. However, a combination of oestrogen and phenylpropanolamine has been shown to help some women (Ahlstrom *et al.* 1990).

SUITABILITY FOR SURGERY

Surgery is the appropriate treatment for genuine stress incontinence but detrusor instability is rarely cured by surgery and, in fact, the symptoms of urgency and frequency of micturition may become worse. Therefore an accurate diagnosis is essential before surgery is undertaken.

Assessment should include history, clinical examination, and the appropriate urodynamic investigations. From the history it is important to ascertain the patient's main complaint and to ask about her urological symptoms, including their severity and duration. Specifically it is important to know about the symptoms of urgency and frequency or if she is experiencing any voiding difficulties. Gynaecological symptoms such as prolapse are also important and any previous pelvic surgery should be noted. A gynaecological examination should include looking at the local tissues for signs of excoriation or atrophy, evaluation of prolapse, and the exclusion of a pelvic mass.

There are no absolute contra-indications to surgery for genuine stress incontinence. There are, however, certain relative contra-indications which include a neurological lesion, a chronic medical condition, or recurrent failed previous surgery. In addition it is probably unwise to operate on women who have not yet completed their family as subsequent pregnancies and deliveries may make the condition recur. Neither age nor obesity should be considered as contra-indications to surgery. Older women have a slightly lower cure rate than younger women but

82   *Treatment*

there is no evidence that the results of surgery in obese women are less good than those in women of normal weight. The final choice must lie with the patient: it is usually unwise to try to persuade her to have an operation if she does not want one.

To know whether or not surgery has been appropriate and successful it is important to carry out pre- and post-operative evaluation which should be both subjective and objective, and to follow up all patients for a minimum of five years. As with any other surgery there is a mortality and a morbidity rate and there may be early or late complications. Side effects include post-operative detrusor instability and voiding difficulties as well as the possibility of immediate failure and later recurrence.

The aims of surgery are to elevate the bladder neck and proximal urethra into an intra-abdominal position where intra-abdominal pressure will act as an additional closing force. Surgery should also support the bladder neck and align it to the postero-superior aspect of the pubic symphysis which will, in some cases, increase outflow resistance.

TYPES OF OPERATION

Numerous different operations have been tried and certainly well over 100 have been described in the literature. Those which are in current usage are shown in Table 6.2.

ANTERIOR COLPORRHAPHY

Anterior colporrhaphy has been used to treat primary genuine stress incontinence in conjunction with a cystourethrocele (Beck and McCormick 1982). Although this procedure is undoubtedly the best operation for anterior vaginal wall prolapse it is certainly not the best operation for genuine stress incontinence. The operative technique involves a longitudinal midline incision down the anterior vaginal wall, the bladder neck is mobilized and one or two Kelly or Pacey sutures are inserted. The pubo-

Table 6.2   Operations for genuine stress incontinence

Vaginal	Anterior colporrhaphy plus buttressing of urethra
	Urethrocliesis
Abdominal	Marshall–Marchetti–Krantz
	Burch colposuspension
Combined	Endoscopic bladder-neck suspension,
	e.g. Stamey (1980), Raz (1984)
	Slings
Complex	Neourethra
	Artificial sphincter
	Urinary diversion

vesical fascia is approximated and the anterior vaginal wall closed. This procedure may be carried out in conjunction with amputation of the cervix (Manchester repair) or with a vaginal hysterectomy.

The complications of anterior colporrhaphy are few, although haemorrhage or trauma to the bladder or urethra may occur. Later problems include recurrent prolapse, urinary incontinence, dyspareunia, or urethral stricture. The results of anterior colporrhaphy have really only been assessed subjectively and follow-up has been poor. However, they are variable, with a cure rate ranging from 40 per cent to 90 per cent. The advantages of an anterior repair are that it is quick and easy to perform with few complications and only a short hospital stay is necessary. It enables a large cystourethrocele to be corrected at the same time but as far as incontinence is concerned, the long-term cure rate is poor.

URETHROCLIESIS

Urethrocliesis is a simple operation and consists of inserting two rows of non-absorbable invaginating sutures along the whole length of the urethra (Frewen 1976). No complications have been reported and approximately 76 per cent of women are cured subjectively. However, this operation is not popular, presumably because the long-term results are poor.

MARSHALL–MARCHETTI–KRANTZ

Marshall–Marchetti–Krantz procedure is used for primary or recurrent genuine stress incontinence (Krantz 1986). A non-absorbable suture material is used to take a double bite of tissue from the bladder neck and hitch it up to the periosteum on the back of the pubic bone. A major complication is osteitis pubis which has been reported to occur in 5 per cent of cases. There may be bladder or urethral injury or haematoma at the time of operation but the main problem is that this operation is unable to correct a cystocele although its results in the treatment of genuine stress incontinence alone are good. Cure rates of up to 96 per cent have been reported.

COLPOSUSPENSION

The colposuspension was originally described by Burch (1961) and has since been modified by many authors. It is used for both primary and recurrent genuine stress incontinence with or without prolapse. The operation is carried out through a transverse suprapubic incision. Retropubic dissection is performed to mobilize the bladder and bladder neck medially off the under-lying fascia and two to four long-term absorbable or non-absorbable sutures are inserted from the para-vaginal fascia to the ileo-pectineal ligament (Fig. 6.3). The complications of this procedure include operative blood loss, urinary tract damage, urinary tract infection, and the later problem of voiding diffi-culties, detrusor instability, and enterocele formation. Urinary tract infection is common but the incidence can be reduced by use of a suprapubic rather than a urethral catheter post-operatively and prophylactic antibiotics should be employed.

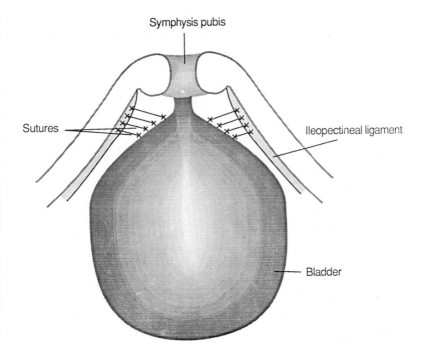

Fig. 6.3 Diagrammatic representation of a colposuspension.

Voiding difficulties are very common and occur in 25 per cent of patients immediately post-operatively. If the pre-operative urodynamic assessment shows a reduced peak flow rate of under 15 ml/s or a maximum voiding pressure of less than 15 cm H_2O then up to 40 per cent of women suffer early voiding difficulties.

Late voiding difficulties occur in approximately 20 per cent of women following colposuspension and are associated with high pre-operative urethral resistance. Detrusor instability has been shown to occur in 18.5 per cent of women at three months following a colposuspension and two-thirds of these women were still symptomatic after five years.

We have recently reviewed the last 100 colposuspensions carried out at King's College Hospital (Cardozo and Cutner

Table 6.3 Success rate of colposuspensions (Cardozo and Cutner 1992)

	Cure rate (per cent)	
	All cases	First operation
Objective	80	84
Subjective	91	94
Objective + subjective	76	81

Table 6.4 Prevalence of detrusor instability resulting from colposuspension (Cardozo and Cutner 1992)

	Detrusor instability (per cent)	
	All cases	First operation
All post-operative cases	14	11
New cases post-operatively	9	5

Table 6.5 Voiding difficulties as a result of colposuspension (Cardozo and Cutner 1992)

	Objective voiding difficulties (per cent)	
	All cases	First operation
Residual > 100 ml	12	11
Peak flow rate (PFR) < 15 ml/s	28	26
Residual > 100 ml + PFR < 15 ml/s	2	3

1992). The women were all treated during 1989 and 1990, using the same technique. They were assessed urodynamically prior to surgery and at 6–12 months post-operatively. Seventy eight were undergoing their first incontinence procedure and the remaining 22 had undergone one or more previous incontinence operations. Table 6.3 shows the cure rate for all patients and for those undergoing their first operation. The only two long-term complications identified were detrusor instability and voiding difficulties and their incidence is shown in Tables 6.4 and 6.5.

A colposuspension type of operation is probably currently the operation of choice for genuine stress incontinence. In all reported series its cure rate is greater than that of the procedures to which it was compared (Table 6.6).

The reasons for failure of the colposuspension have been evaluated, and lower cure rates occur in those women with pre-operative co-existent detrusor instability, older women, women who have undergone previous incontinence surgery, and women who have a low maximum urethral closure pressure (less than 25 cm H_2O).

ENDOSCOPIC BLADDER-NECK SUSPENSION

Endoscopic bladder-neck suspensions are indicated for primary or recurrent genuine stress incontinence and some authors have advocated their use in the very old or frail. They are easier to perform in a surgically difficult pelvis where recurrent surgery has lead to scarring, as they do not require any open dissection. Various techniques have been described (Pereyra and Lebherz 1978; Stamey 1980; Raz 1984), but all utilize two nylon sutures passed 'blind' from the para-vaginal fascia to the rectus sheath or vice versa (Fig. 6.4). The complication rate is small although infection of the 'buffers' has been a problem in some cases. Urinary tract damage may occur and some women complain of post-operative urgency. Although there have been some reports of a high cure rate, other studies are less encouraging. These differences are probably due to the mode of evaluation and length of follow-up.

Table 6.6 Cure rates of incontinence operations compared with colposuspension

	Colposuspension	Anterior repair	Pereyra	Stamey
Stanton and Cardozo (1979)	85 per cent ($n = 25$)	36 per cent ($n = 25$)		40 per cent ($n = 25$)
Mundy (1983)	73 per cent ($n = 26$)			
Weil et al. (1984)	91 per cent ($n = 34$)	57 per cent ($n = 30$)	50 per cent ($n = 22$)	
Bhatia and Bergman (1985)	98 per cent ($n = 44$)		85 per cent ($n = 20$)	
Bergman et al. (1989)	87 per cent ($n = 101$)	69 per cent ($n = 99$)	70 per cent ($n = 98$)	

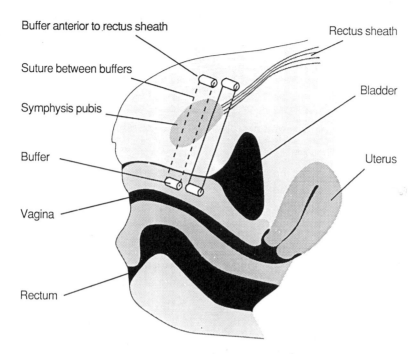

Buffer anterior to rectus sheath

Suture between buffers

Symphysis pubis

Buffer

Vagina

Rectum

Rectus sheath

Bladder

Uterus

Fig. 6.4 Diagrammatic representation of the Stamey procedure.

Endoscopic bladder-neck suspensions are advantageous because they are quick and easy to perform. A general anaesthetic does not necessarily need to be employed, as regional block is quite adequate. They only involve a short hospital stay and a few centres have advocated endoscopic bladder-neck suspension as a day-case procedure. Complications are few, although there is some evidence to suggest that they do not produce a high long-term objective cure rate.

SLINGS

Sling procedures are indicated for recurrent rather than primary genuine stress incontinence. Many different types have been

described. They can be performed using either organic material
(bovine rectus sheath or strips of the patient's own rectus sheath)
or inorganic material (Marlex, Mersilene, Gore-tex or Silastic).
The sling can be either inserted via an abdominal incision with
retropubic dissection, or through a vaginal incision. More often,
however, a combined approach is used. The sling is passed between the bladder neck and vaginal skin (Fig. 6.5) and is
anchored either to the rectus sheath or to the ileo-pectineal
ligament.

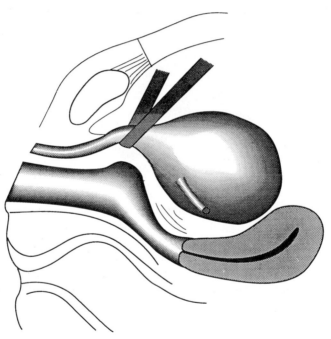

Fig. 6.5 Diagrammatic representation of a sling operation.

Complication rates are high and include haemorrhage, infection, injury to the bladder or urethra, erosion of the sling into
the urethra, and a very significant incidence of post-operative
voiding difficulties both immediate and long term. The results of

slings have been assessed in various different studies and cure rates of up to 95 per cent are claimed (Fianu and Soderberg 1983). However, in most studies the patients were not homogeneous and they have been assessed subjectively rather than objectively and only for a short period of time post-operatively.

The advantage of sling procedures is that they are useful when the urethra is scarred or the vagina is narrowed. However, they function by causing outflow obstruction and patients who are going to undergo a sling procedure need to realize that they may require clean, intermittent self-catheterization, possibly indefinitely.

INJECTABLES

Because of the problem of treating women who have a fixed, scarred (drain-pipe) urethra, various substances have been injected around the bladder neck to produce relative outflow obstruction. Teflon was originally tried with reasonably successful results. However, there have been problems with migration of Teflon to the lung and brain. More recently Gax (glutaraldehyde cross-linked bovine) collagen has been evaluated and early results appear to be encouraging (Appell *et al.* 1989). This treatment works by causing obstruction, but although poor flow rates have been demonstrated post-operatively, the incidence of significant urinary retention seems to be remarkably low. As yet this technique has not been adequately evaluated and there need to be more studies which include a follow-up period.

NEOURETHRA

For those women who have failed multiple previous operations several complex procedures exist. The neo-urethra is useful in cases of congenital abnormality or where there has been severe trauma. An anterior flap of bladder is raised and reconstructed as a tube to form a new urethra. The complication rate is high with fistula, stricture formation, and failure of the technique (Tanagho 1986).

ARTIFICIAL SPHINCTERS

Artificial sphincters are now in regular use, especially in North America, and are indicated in cases of recurrent genuine stress incontinence where there is a rigid scarred urethra, or in cases of mixed incontinence due to congenital abnormalities. The operation involves the insertion of a fluid-filled cuff which is placed around the bladder neck and connected to a deflation pump which is sited in the left labium majus. The system is connected to an intra-peritoneal balloon reservoir. Voiding occurs after the cuff has been deflated and continence is maintained by the obstruction caused by the inflated cuff. The complication rate is high but the main problem is that these devices are exceedingly expensive. Bladder or urethral injury may occur during insertion but if this occurs the device can be de-activated initially and re-activated when any damage has healed. If the cuff becomes infected the result may be disastrous and the whole device has to be removed. Cuff erosion occurs through the urethra and into the vagina particularly when the tissues are scarred after multiple previous operations and these devices are prone to mechanical faults. The application of artificial sphincters is not yet clear but hopefully in the future they will become less expensive and less complex (Furlow 1986).

CHOICE OF OPERATION

Under normal circumstances the choice of operation will be decided by the experience and preference of the operator. A colposuspension is the most likely to produce a lasting cure in primary or recurrent genuine stress incontinence and will correct a cystocele at the same time. Endoscopic bladder-neck suspensions are less arduous and can be combined with an anterior colporrhaphy in order to reduce a cystocele at the same time. Sling procedures are useful only when the vagina is narrowed and scarred, and they have a high complication rate, but in the future injectables may be the answer for this type of woman.

HOW MAY WE IMPROVE THE RESULTS OF INCONTINENCE SURGERY?

Pre-operatively, it is important to suggest that women stop smoking and therefore improve any chronic chest disease; any other medical condition should be treated appropriately. Oestrogen therapy for post-menopausal women may improve the tissues and peri-operative physiotherapy to the pelvic floor should be advocated. There is no evidence that the results of surgery are worse in obese women but there is certainly a greater morbidity, and surgery is more difficult. These obese women should be encouraged to lose weight although not as a prerequisite to an operation.

During the course of the operation it is important to pay particular attention to the number of sutures that are used and the suture material. Approximation of the tissues is important and peri-operative antibiotics will reduce the incidence of infection. A suction drain should be used to reduce haematoma formation and a suprapubic catheter is associated with a reduced urinary tract infection rate and a shorter time to spontaneous voiding. Post-operatively it is essential to investigate all cases of failed surgery and also to follow patients up for a reasonable length of time in order to know what the recurrence rate is.

Finally, it is important to remember that all surgery carries a mortality and morbidity rate whereas urinary incontinence does not. In addition, as the first operation is the most likely to cure the condition, the best operation should be chosen for the first attempt.

REFERENCES

Ahlstrom, K., Sandahl, B., Sjoberg, B., Ulmsten, U., Stormby, N., and Lindskog, M. (1990). Effect of combined treatment with phenyl-propanolamine and estriol, compared to estriol treatment alone, in postmenopausal women with stress urinary incontinence. *Gynecol. Obstet. Invest.*, **30**, 37–43.

Appell, R.A., Goodman, J.R., McGuire, E.J., Wang, S.C., Bennett, A.H., DeRidder, P.A., and Webster, G.D. (1989). Multicenter study of periurethral and transurethral Gax-collagen injection for urinary incontinence. Proceedings of the 19th Annual Meeting of the International Continence Society, Ljubliana, 1989. *Neurourol. Urodyn.*, **8**, 339–40.

Beck, P.R. and McCormick, S. (1982). Treatment of urinary stress incontinence with anterior colporrhaphy. *Obstet. Gynecol.*, **59**, 269–74.

Bergman, A., Koonings, P.P., and Ballard, C.A. (1989). Primary stress urinary incontinence and pelvic relaxation: prospective randomized comparison of three different operations. *Am. J. Obstet. Gynecol.*, **161**, 97–101.

Bhatia, N.N. and Bergman, A. (1985). Modified Burch retropubic urethropexy versus modified Pereyra procedure for stress urinary incontinence. *Obstet. Gynecol.*, **66**, 255–61.

Burch, J. (1961). Urethrovaginal fixation to Cooper's ligament for correction of stress incontinence, cystocele and prolapse. *Am. J. Obstet. Gynecol.*, **81**, 281–90.

Cardozo, L.D. (1990). The role of estrogen in the treatment of female urinary incontinence. *J. Am. Geriatr. Soc.*, **38**, 326–8.

Cardozo, L.D. and Cutner, A. (1992). Surgical management of genuine stress incontinence. *Contemporary Reviews in Obstetrics and Gynaecology*, **4**, 36–41.

Fianu, S. and Soderberg, G. (1983). Absorbable polyglactin mesh for retropubic sling operations in female urinary stress incontinence. *Gynecol. Obstet. Invest.*, **16**, 45–50.

Frewen, W.K. (1976) Urethral graft in stress incontinence. In *Communications to the Sixth Annual Congress, 1976*. International Continence Society, Antwerp.

Furlow, W.L. (1986). Artificial sphincter. In *Surgery of female incontinence* (ed. S.L. Stanton and E.A. Tanagho) (2nd edn), pp. 155–73. Springer, Berlin.

Kegel, A.H. (1949). The physiologic treatment of poor tone and function of the genital muscles and of urinary stress incontinence. *West. J. Surg. Obstet. Gynecol.*, **57**, 527–35.

Krantz, E.K. (1986). The Marshall–Marchetti–Krantz procedure. In *Surgery of female incontinence* (ed. S.L. Stanton and E.A. Tanagho) (2nd edn), pp. 87–93. Springer, Berlin.

Laycock, J. (1988). Interferential therapy in the treatment of genuine stress incontinence. In *Proc. 18th Annual Meeting of the International Continence Society*, Oslo, pp. 265–6.

Mundy, A.R. (1983). A trial comparing the Stamey bladder neck suspension procedure with colposuspension for the treatment of stress incontinence. *Br. J. Urol.*, **55**, 687–90.

Peattie, A.B., Plevnik, S., and Stanton, S.L. (1988). Vaginal cones: a conservative method of treating genuine stress incontinence. *Br. J. Obstet. Gynaecol.*, **95**, 1049–53.

Pereyra, A.J. and Lebherz, T.B. (1978). The revised Pereyra procedure. In *Gynecologic and Obstetric Urology* (ed. H.J. Buchsbaum and J.D. Schmidt), pp. 208–22. Saunders, Philadelphia.

Raz, S. (ed.) (1984). Needle urethral–vesical suspension procedures. In *Female urology*, pp. 276–83. Saunders, Philadelphia.

Shepherd, A.M. and Montgomery, E. (1983). Treatment of genuine stress incontinence with a new perineometer. *Physiotherapy*, **69**, 113.

Stamey, T.A. (1980). Endoscopic suspension of the bladder neck for urinary incontinence in females: report of 203 consecutive cases. *Ann. Surg.*, **192**, 465–71.

Stanton, S.L. and Cardozo, L. (1979). A comparison of vaginal and suprapubic surgery in the correction of incontinence due to urethral sphincter incompetence. *Br. J. Urol.*, **51**, 497–9.

Tanagho, E.A. (1986). Neourethra: rationale, surgical technique and indications. In *Surgery of female incontinence* (ed. S.L. Stanton and E.A. Tanagho) (2nd edn), pp. 145–53. Springer, Berlin.

Weil, A., Reyes, H., Bischoff, P., Rottenberg, R.D., and Krauer, F. (1984). Modifications of the urethral resting and stress profiles after different types of surgery for urinary stress incontinence. *Br. J. Obstet, Gynaecol.*, **91**, 46–55.

7

Detrusor instability

INTRODUCTION

Women with mild or intermittent symptoms may only require reassurance and simple measures such as decreased fluid intake, avoidance of tea, coffee, and alcohol, or a change in voiding habits. The majority, however, will require further treatment. The methods used attempt either to improve central control, as in behavioural intervention, or to alter detrusor innervation using drugs or surgical techniques. Only if these measures fail are procedures employed which do not treat the instability but act to increase the size of the reservoir.

SPECIFIC TREATMENTS

The therapeutic options currently employed include the following:

(1) drug therapy;
(2) behavioural therapy;
(3) maximal electrical stimulation;
(4) phenol injections;
(5) augmentation cystoplasty.

Many other surgical forms of treatment have been tried in the past including vaginal denervation, selective sacral neurectomy, cystodistension, and bladder transection. All have been reported to be efficacious initially, but due to high complication rates or long-term relapse, have been superseded.

DRUG THERAPY

Pharmacotherapy is still required for the successful treatment of
most patients with detrusor instability. Drugs may be subdivided
into groups according to their pharmacological mode of action.
These are shown in Table 7.1.

Table 7.1 Drugs used in the treatment of detrusor instability

Drug	Anticholinergic	Direct relaxant	Dose
Propantheline	*		15–90 mg qds
Oxybutynin	*	*	2.5–10 mg bd/tds
Imipramine	*	Also has central action	50 mg bd (up to 150 mg in a single dose)
DDAVP	Reduces urine production		20–40 mg nocte (nasal spray)
Oestrogens	Raise sensory threshold of bladder		

Anticholinergic agents

Since the parasympathetic nervous system is mediated by acetylcholine, anti-muscarinic drugs such as atropine are of use in the
treatment of detrusor instability. Its lack of specificity, however,
makes atropine unacceptable because of the systemic side effects
of dry mouth, blurred vision, tachycardia, drowsiness, and
constipation.

Propantheline (Probanthine) is a related drug with fewer side
effects (Blaivas *et al.* 1980). It is a quaternary ammonium analogue of atropine with both anti-muscarinic and anti-nicotinic
properties which acts at both the ganglionic level and at the

neuromuscular junction. When given orally in a dose of 15 mg four times per day (qds) it is often ineffective. The dose may therefore be increased as high as 90 mg qds, but slowly to minimize side effects. Gastrointestinal absorption is aided by taking the drug before meals. Propantheline is a cheap drug, with few side effects, and is particularly useful when frequency of micturition is a major problem.

Emepronium carageenate is a drug which has similar properties to propantheline. It is derived from seaweed and is currently marketed in Europe, but not in the United Kingdom.

Musculotropic relaxants

Oxybutynin (Cystrin, Ditropan) is probably the most effective drug available. It has a direct spasmolytic effect as well as anticholinergic properties. However, the dose used must be balanced with the patients ability to tolerate the dry mouth, throat, and lingering bad taste which accompany its therapeutic effect. It is a drug with a short half-life, and therefore it is rapidly effective following ingestion. A dose may be taken as prophylaxis to control symptoms for short periods, e.g. while shopping or at the cinema. The standard dosage is 5 mg orally twice daily but this may be increased up to 10 mg three times a day (Cardozo *et al.* 1987). An alternative dose regimen of 3 mg three times a day has been advocated, and appears to maintain reasonable efficacy, whilst the incidence of side effects resulting in discontinuation of therapy is reduced (Moore *et al.* 1990). Patients should be encouraged to titrate the dosage themselves to find their own acceptable pattern of administration.

Flavoxate (Urispas) is a tertiary amine which inibits phosphodiesterase, resulting in raised levels of cyclic AMP, which leads to muscle relaxation. It also has analgesic and local anaesthetic properties. Commonly prescribed in a dose of 200 mg three times per day (tds), it is poorly absorbed from the gut, and doubt has been cast as to its true efficacy in the treatment of detrusor instability. Its effects may be no superior to those of placebo. Terflavoxate is a newly developed drug which is a derivative of flavoxate. Its efficacy in the treatment of detrusor instability has not been evaluated.

Calcium channel blockers

Until 1991, Terodiline was the most widely prescribed drug in the United Kingdom for the treatment of detrusor instability. It has been withdrawn by its manufacturer, due to the association of its use with the incidence of a ventricular tachyarrhythmia, *torsades de pointes*.

It acted on the detrusor by limiting the availability of calcium ions required for smooth muscle contraction, and also had intrinsic anticholinergic effects (Tapp *et al*. 1987). It had a long half-life and therefore accumulation was likely to occur, especially in the elderly. Terodiline was of undoubted benefit to many women with detrusor instability and its withdrawal reduces the therapeutic options now available. Oxybutynin is the most efficacious alternative drug therapy.

Other drugs which decrease contractility

Imipramine is an analogue of chlorpromazine and is commonly used as an antidepressant agent. It acts by inhibiting reuptake of noradrenaline and 5-hydroxytryptamine into the presynaptic membrane, and thus potentiates their action. This may result in bladder relaxation and also increase outlet resistance. It also has anticholinergic and local anaesthetic properties. Imipramine sometimes causes the common anticholinergic side effects as well as tremor, sedation, and convulsions. If treatment is stopped abruptly, withdrawal reactions may occur involving nausea, vomiting and malaise. ECG changes have been reported, including tachycardia, atrial flutter, atrial fibrillation, ventricular flutter, and both atrioventricular and interventricular block.

Imipramine is, however, a most useful drug for the treatment of nocturia and nocturnal enuresis (Castleden *et al*. 1981). A dose of up to 150 mg may be given safely, but the standard

dosage is 50 mg twice daily (bd). Imipramine given prophylactic-
ally before sexual intercourse may be of benefit to patients with
coital incontinence at orgasm.

Anti-diuretic drugs

1-Desamino-8-D arginine vasopressin (DDAVP) is a long-acting
synthetic analogue of vasopressin, and is a peptide hormone
containing eight amino acids. DDAVP can be administered
intranasally and is effective for 12–24 h, having a half-life of
75 minutes due to slow metabolic clearance. Whilst it has full
antidiuretic potency and increases permeability in the distal
convoluted tubules and collecting ducts of the kidney, unlike
vasopressin it has no significant effect on blood pressure. It has
a lesser effect on smooth muscle contraction and so pallor, colic,
bronchospasm, and coronary artery or uterine spasm do not
occur.

DDAVP is a useful drug in the treatment of nocturia and
nocturnal enuresis, and acts by reducing urine output during
sleep (Hilton and Stanton 1982). Because the bladder fills more
slowly, and the total volume of urine is reduced, the unstable
bladder is less likely to contract. Some patients with nocturia or
nocturnal enuresis have abnormal patterns of ADH release
which can be treated successfully with DDAVP. It has been
shown to be safe for long-term use, but caution must be used
when treating patients with coronary artery disease, hypertension, heart failure, or epilepsy (Knudsen *et al.* 1989).

Hormone replacement therapy

No studies have shown that oestrogen therapy improves incontinence due to detrusor instability. Oestrogen deficiency following
the menopause causes changes in all layers of the urethra which
has abundant oestrogen receptors. The bladder itself possesses
fewer receptors. Sensory urgency is, however, improved by
oestrogen therapy, which is thought to raise the sensory
threshold of the bladder (Fantl *et al.* 1988).

Summary

Drugs may be used alone or in combination. Propantheline and imipramine can be used together for the treatment of diurnal and nocturnal frequency. In a similar way, DDAVP may be used in combination with oxybutynin. Drugs may be used in conjunction with other forms of treatment, e.g. bladder retraining. The choice of drug for each patient depends on their predominant symptoms and their tolerance of side effects.

BEHAVIOURAL THERAPY

This type of treatment is based on the premise that learning is the most important determinant of behaviour, and that behaviour can be altered as a result of experience. Thus human behaviour is seen as a collection of responses to specific situations. Detrusor instability, in some instances, is viewed as a result of maladaptive learned behaviour. Treatment is aimed at either 'unlearning' maladaptive behaviour or relearning a more appropriate one.

Bladder drill

This treatment was first referred to as bladder discipline (Jeffcoate and Francis 1966), and was popularized by Frewen (1978). A regimen of timed voiding is employed on either an out-patient or an in-patient basis. The time between voids is gradually increased over a period of days. High success rates are reported for in-patient bladder drill, but the rate of relapse in the long term is high. The regimen suggested by Jarvis (1981) is commonly employed and is shown below.

1. Exclude pathology and admit to hospital.
2. Explain rationale to patient.
3. Instruct to void every one and a half hours during the day. She must not void between these times; she must wait or be incontinent.

4. Increase voiding interval by half an hour when initial goal achieved, and continue with two-hourly voiding, etc.
5. Normal fluid intake.
6. Keep fluid balance chart.
7. Encouragement from nursing and medical staff.

Bladder drill is particularly useful for elderly patients, in whom it has been shown to be more efficacious than drug therapy. It also avoids the potential risks and side effects of pharmacotherapy. In practice, a combination of anticholinergic therapy and bladder drill is often used with good effect.

Biofeedback

This involves the use of electronic equipment to monitor a normally unconscious physiological process, and to convey this information to the individual so that a change in a particular direction may be brought about (Cardozo *et al.* 1978). The information is fedback as an audible, tactile, or visual signal. This type of treatment requires a great deal of input from motivated doctors or nurses.

Hypnotherapy and acupuncture

Other forms of behavioural therapy, including hypnotherapy (Freeman and Baxby 1982) and acupuncture (Philip *et al.* 1988) have been reported as successful in the treatment of detrusor instability. Few controlled trials of such intervention have been conducted, and much of the symptomatic benefit may be due to a placebo effect. Both hypnosis and acupuncture require a high level of specialist skill and are unavailable as routine treatments on the NHS.

Acupuncture is thought to act by increasing levels of endorphins and enkephalins in the cerebrospinal fluid. Enkephalins inhibit detrusor contractility *in vitro*. Naloxone, an opiate antagonist, conversely causes decreased bladder capacity and increased detrusor pressures. Recently, infrared low-power laser has been used on acupuncture points, with similar efficacy to the traditional Chinese method.

Bladder drill, biofeedback, and hypnotherapy have all been reported as having a cure/improvement rate of approximately 80 per cent in the short term.

MAXIMAL ELECTRICAL STIMULATION

This technique involves stimulation of the pelvic floor musculature using vaginal or rectal plug electrodes. Stimulation of pudendal nerve afferent fibres leads to inhibition of efferent motor impulses to the bladder and results in the abolition of spontaneous detrusor contractions. Objective success rates of 77 per cent have been reported up to one year following short-term maximal electrical stimulation (Plevnik *et al.* 1986). Daily treatment sessions lasting 20 minutes are continued for 30 days. The electrode is connected to a battery-powered unit which provides a stimulus with a frequency of 20 Hz, pulse duration of 0.1 ms and a variable current of 0–90 mA. The patient is taught to increase the stimulus strength to just below the level of discomfort. This technique is promising and requires further evaluation.

SURGICAL TECHNIQUES

Historically, many different surgical procedures have been utilized but few have stood the test of time.

Vaginal denervation, bladder transection, and sacral neurectomy were techniques aimed at permanently disrupting the motor supply to the detrusor. Each procedure had a limited effect and was associated with unacceptable complications.

Bladder distension, which was originally introduced as a treatment for carcinoma of the bladder (Helmstein 1972), became a popular method of treatment. Several subsequent studies have shown it to be of limited efficacy, with a high rate of complications, notably bladder rupture. The following operative procedures, however, are of value in selected cases of detrusor instability.

Transvesical phenol injections

Transvesical blockade of nerve plexuses adjacent to the bladder has been described using a 25 cm long needle passed down the side channel of a cystoscope. The tip is introduced mid-way between the ureteric orifice and the bladder neck and is advanced 2–3 cm. Ten millilitres of 6 per cent aqueous phenol is then injected. The procedure is performed bilaterally.

Good results have been reported in women with detrusor hyperreflexia (Blackford *et al.* 1984). It has been suggested that there is a role for phenol injections in patients with an indwelling catheter and detrusor hyperreflexia who have problems with bypassing due to detrusor contractions. One set of injections may give relief of symptoms and avoid a lifetime of drug therapy.

There is a recognized incidence of urinary retention requiring intermittent self-catheterization of about 8 per cent. Other complications include sciatic nerve palsy, ureteric sloughing, and vesico-vaginal fistula.

More recent studies do not confirm these good results, and for patients with idiopathic detrusor instability only 25 per cent derive any short-term benefit. Very little benefit is maintained beyond one year following treatment. For these patients, the temporary nature of any improvement does not warrant the risk of anaesthesia. They may be better treated by augmentation cystoplasty (Rosenbaum *et al.* 1988).

Augmentation cystoplasty

Some patients will not respond to any medical intervention or find their side effects too incapacitating. They may have been subjected to cystodistension or phenol injections, as these are still relatively commonly performed procedures. If symptoms are still severe, augmentation cystoplasty should be considered. The operation involves bisecting the bladder in a coronal plane anterior to the ureteric orifices to within 1 cm of the bladder neck. The distance is measured and a corresponding length of ileum is isolated, opened along its anti-mesenteric border, and sutured as a patch into the defect. This segment is thought to act by absorbing, and thereby reducing, the effect of unstable detrusor contractions.

A cure rate of up to 90 per cent has been reported by several authors (Mundy and Stephenson 1985). There is a significant risk of post-operative voiding difficulties, possibly as a result of diminished voiding pressures, caused by the presence of the ileal segment. This may be overcome by performing a sphincterotomy or by teaching the patient clean intermittent self-catheterization. Less common complications such as urine leakage from the anastomosis remove, requiring revision, and small-bowel obstruction have been described.

Mucus production by the bowel segment occasionally causes distress to the patient who may have to strain to pass mucus plugs. Ingestion of 200 ml of cranberry juice a day helps to reduce mucus viscidity.

The chronic exposure of the ileal mucosa to urine has given cause for concern with regard to possible malignant change. There is a five per cent risk of adenocarcinoma arising in ureterosigmoidostomies, where colonic mucosa is exposed to the N-nitrosamines found in both urine and faeces. Biopsies of the ileal segment taken from patients with 'clam cystoplasties' show evidence of chronic inflammation and villous atrophy. In bilharzia, chronic inflammation is thought to predispose to carcinoma which is associated with this condition.

There have been reports of cases of adenocarcinoma arising in the ileal segment. In three cases, occurring in patients seven, twenty-two, and twenty-four years following surgery, all three had initially had tuberculosis as a cause of their symptoms; all had been troubled with recurrent urinary tract infections, and had high residual urine volumes post-operatively. It is clear therefore that patients undergoing augmentation cystoplasty require long-term follow-up.

REFERENCES

Blackford, W., Murray, K., Stephenson, T.P., and Mundy, A.R. (1984). Results of transvesical infiltration of the pelvis with phenol in 116 patients. *Br. J. Urol.*, **56**, 647–9.

Blaivas, J.G., Labib, K.B., Michalik, S.J., and Zayed, A.A.H. (1980). Cystometric response to propantheline in detrusor hyperreflexia: therapeutic implications. *J. Urol.*, **124**, 259–62.

Cardozo, L.D., Abrams, P.H., Stanton, S.L., and Feneley, R.C.L. (1978). Idiopathic bladder instability treated by biofeedback. *Br. J. Urol.*, **50**, 521–3.

Cardozo, L.D., Cooper, D.J., and Versi, E. (1987). Oxybutynin chloride in the management of idiopathic detrusor instability. *Neurourol. Urodyn.*, **6**, 88–9.

Castleden, C.M., George, C.F., Renwick, A.G., and Asher, M.J. (1981). Imipramine, a possible alternative to current therapy for urinary incontinence in the elderly. *J. Urol.*, **125**, 318–20.

Fantl, J.A., Wyman, J.F., Anderson, R.L., Matt, D.W., and Bump, R.C. (1988). Postmenopausal urinary incontinence: comparison between non-oestrogen supplemented and oestrogen supplemented women. *Obstet. Gynecol.*, **71**, 823–8.

Freeman, R.M. and Baxby, K. (1982). Hypnotherapy for incontinence caused by the unstable bladder. *Br. Med. J.*, **284**, 1831–4.

Frewen, W.K. (1978). An objective assessment of the unstable bladder of psychological origin. *Br.J. Urol.*, **50**, 246–9.

Helmstein, K. (1972). Treatment of bladder carcinoma by a hydrostatic pressure technique. *Br. J. Urol.*, **44**, 434–50.

Hilton, P. and Stanton, S.L. (1982). The use of desmopressin (DDAVP) in nocturnal urine frequency in the female. *Br. J. Urol.*, **54**, 252–5.

Jarvis, G.J. (1981). A controlled trial of bladder drill and drug therapy in the management of detrusor instability. *Br. J. Urol.*, **53**, 565–6.

Jeffcoate, T.N.A. and Francis, W.J.A. (1966). Urgency incontinence in the female. *Am. J. Obstet. Gynecol.*, **94**, 604–18.

Knudsen, U.B., Rittig, S., Pederen, J.B., Norgaard, J.P., and Djaarhus, J.C. (1989). Long term treatment of nocturnal enuresis with desmopressin—influence on urinary output and haematological parameters. *Neurol. Urodynam.*, **8**, 348–9.

Moore, K.H., Hay, D.M., Imrie, A.E., Watson, A., and Goldstein, M. (1990). Oxybutynin hydrochloride (3 mg) in the treatment of women with idiopathic detrusor instability. *Br. J. Urol.*, **66**, 479–85.

Mundy, A.R. and Stephenson, T.P. (1985). 'Clam' ileocystoplasty for the treatment of refractory urge incontinence. *Br. J. Urol.*, **57**, 641–6.

Philip, T., Shah, P.J.R., and Worth, P.H.L. (1988). Acupuncture in the treatment of bladder instability. *Br. J. Urol.*, **61**, 490–3.

Plevnik, S., Janez, J., Vrtacnik, P., Trasinar, B., and Vodusek, D.B. (1986). Short term electrical stimulation: home treatment for urinary incontinence. *World J. Urol.*, **4**, 24–6.

Rosenbaum, T.P., Shah, P.J.R., and Worth, P.H.L. (1988). Transtrigonal phenol: the end of an era? *Neurourol. Urodynam.*, **7**, 294–5.

Tapp, A.J.S., Fall, M., Norgaard, J., Massey, A., Choa, R., Carr, T., Korhonen, M., and Abrams, P. (1987). A dose titrated multicentre study of terodiline in the treatment of detrusor instability. In *Proc. 17th Annual Meeting of the International Continence Society, Bristol.*

8

Voiding difficulties and overflow incontinence

INTRODUCTION

Voiding difficulties can be due to a hypotonic detrusor or outflow obstruction, or the two causes may coexist. Initial assessment is essential and should include a careful history of the presenting symptoms and present medication and appropriate urodynamic investigations. In addition, in some cases renal function will require investigation as it may be compromised.

GENERAL MEASURES

Mild cases of voiding difficuties may require no treatment at all. Drugs with anticholinergic side effects should be withdrawn where possible. If the woman merely complains of frequency or recurrent urinary tract infections due to a chronic post-micturition residual of urine, double voiding may alleviate the problem. For this the woman is taught to completely empty her bladder each time she passes urine by attempting to void a second time a few minutes after she feels that voiding is complete.

In those cases where voiding difficulties follow operations for incontinence, a change in voiding position may help the bladder to empty completely. Operations for genuine stress incontinence alter the angle of the urethra and may make it necessary to adopt a more upright position during voiding to enable the bladder to empty completely. Recurrent urinary tract infections may be prevented by the use of long-term prophylactic antibiotics. A trial of urethral dilatation for all cases of voiding difficulty may result in stress incontinence due to damage of the urethral sphincter mechanism and is therefore undesirable.

DETRUSOR HYPOTONIA

In cases where there has been a recent episode of acute retention of urine, the bladder will require initial rest. This is achieved by use of a catheter on free drainage which may be required for a period of a few weeks. A suprapubic catheter is preferable as it is associated with a lower incidence of urinary tract infection and resumption of voiding can be monitored by clamping the catheter and measuring post-micturition urinary residuals.

An alternative is to teach the woman clean, intermittent self-catheterization which she performs after each void, measuring the residual on each occasion (Webb *et al.* 1990). Once the residual is less than 100 ml, the procedure can be stopped.

Chronic voiding difficulties due to a hypotonic detrusor may be helped by cholinergic agents. These drugs will directly stimulate the detrusor muscle. A subcutaneous injection of carbachol 250 mg will cause immediate contraction of the detrusor and can be used as a diagnostic test to assess the possible success of long-term oral therapy. Oral therapy consists of bethanecol in a starting dose of 25 mg tds. Response to treatment should be monitored by the measurement of post-micturition urinary residuals.

Some women with mild voiding difficulties may merely complain of nocturia as the functional bladder capacity is not adequate to last the night. These women are successfully treated with decreased fluid intake in the evening combined with intermittent self-catheterization once before going to bed each night.

In many cases where the problem is long standing and there is little or no detrusor function, the only treatment is long-term clean intermittent self-catheterization. This is preferable to a permanent indwelling catheter as the incidence of urinary tract infections is lower and the lifestyle more normal.

Outflow obstruction

This is treated by removing the cause of obstruction. It is important to adequately investigate the cause as a pelvic mass may need to be removed and in such a case surgery to the urethra would be inappropriate. Where a urethral stricture is the cause, a urethrotomy should be carried out. This is preferable to urethral dilatation as the latter has a high recurrence rate and repeated dilatations may damage the urethral sphincter mechanism or cause urethral fibrosis. Either an otis urethrotomy or a urethrotomy under cystoscopic guidance is performed with three incisions along the whole length of the urethra. Post-operatively a large-bore urethral catheter (at least 18 French) should be left *in situ* for 7–10 days. Urethrotomy is not without complications and prior investigation is essential to ensure that urethral outflow obstruction is the cause of the voiding difficulties.

Failed cases

Where the detrusor fails to respond to cholinergic therapy or there is a scarred urethra, the primary pathology cannot be cured. In the past these women were treated with a permanent indwelling catheter but nowadays long-term clean intermittent self-catheterization is preferable. This, however, relies upon good patient motivation, adequate teaching, and a modicum of manual dexterity.

REFERENCE

Webb, R.J., Lawson, A.L., and Neal, D.E. (1990). Clean intermittent self-catheterisation in 172 adults. *Br. J. Urol.*, **65**, 20–3.

9

The management of urinary fistulae

The early management of a vesico-vaginal fistula depends on the underlying cause and the duration of the abnormality. Surgical trauma, if recognized, may be repaired within 24 h. However, most fistulae present between 4 and 21 days, when avascular necrosis occurs. A period of continuous urethral catheterization is worthwhile, provided that most of the urine drains via this route, since the defect may close spontaneously over a period of six weeks with appropriate antibiotic cover. If there is tissue loss following an obstetric slough injury, then bladder drainage and antibiotic treatment should be instituted. Faecal contamination due to damage to the rectum may require defunctioning colostomy prior to definitive repair. It is essential that tissue loss has ceased and infection is controlled prior to surgical repair. This may mean a delay of up to three months in cases of obstetric fistulae. Associated problems of skin excoriation, urinary tract infection, anaemia, electrolyte imbalance, and possible uraemia should be dealt with at this stage. Some people advocate early closure of gynaecological fistulae, but most defer surgery. Ureteric injury should be dealt with immediately, even if only by nephrostomy to protect renal function.

The route of repair may be vaginal or abdominal depending on ease of access. Bladder and urethral fistulae are best treated vaginally, whereas involvement of the ureters or bowel may necessitate an abdominal approach. The use of a pedicle graft which provides viable tissue may be required if tissue loss is extensive. A Martius graft (subcutaneous fat pedicle from the labium majus) or a gracilis graft may be used for this purpose.

Post-operatively, free bladder drainage is continued for two weeks but longer for fistula secondary to irradiation. Complications of surgery include clot retention and catheter blockage. This requires prompt treatment to prevent breakdown of the suture line of repair. Overall success rates for primary closure of surgical fistulae should be over 90 per cent. For obstetric fistulae in the developing world the figures are 75 per cent with a further 15 per cent closed following a second procedure. Results of post-irradiation fistula repair are less successful with cure rates as low as 60 per cent. Urinary diversion should only be performed as a last resort, and implantation of ureters into bowel must only be undertaken if there is no recto-vaginal fistula and the anal sphincter is capable of maintaining continence of liquid faeces.

IV

Difficult problems

10

Dispelling myths

There are many, commonly held misconceptions concerning urinary incontinence. The following statements have been made repeatedly, by both patients and professionals attending our urodynamic unit. By stating established facts, we hope to clear up areas of misunderstanding and spread the truth, in order to improve education and allay anxiety.

'URINARY INCONTINENCE IS NORMAL'

Involuntary loss of urine is never normal. In certain situations it may be short-lived (e.g. during or immediately following pregnancy) or self-limiting. However, persistent symptoms indicate pathology and warrant investigation and appropriate treatment.

'INCONTINENCE ONLY AFFECTS THE ELDERLY'

Urinary incontinence may affect women of any age. Genuine stress incontinence has a peak prevalence in the 40–50 years age group whereas detrusor instability is more prevalent in the very young and very old. The impact of incontinence on the quality of life of an individual will depend on many factors including age, but age alone should not dictate patient management. All women with urinary incontinence require thorough assessment.

'NOTHING CAN BE DONE TO HELP'

On the contrary, most cases of urinary incontinence may be cured or significantly improved, once the cause has been diagnosed and treated. Advice on simple measures to alleviate symptoms is available from general practitioners, district nurses, and continence advisors. However, referral at an early stage for urodynamic investigation may reduce treatment failures and disillusionment among patients.

'IT ALL STARTED AFTER MY BABY WAS BORN'

This is a very common claim which is often difficult to verify. Many women experience urinary symptoms for the first time during pregnancy, and these may persist following the birth of the baby. This may be perceived by the mother as a direct result of delivery rather than of the pregnancy as a whole. Urinary incontinence may arise directly as a result of pudendal nerve and pelvic floor damage following labour, but evidence suggests that a proportion of women develop detrusor instability during pregnancy which may persist following delivery. If urinary incontinence persists after the puerperium, then urodynamic investigation is indicated.

'INCONTINENCE RUNS IN MY FAMILY'

Apart from rare forms of muscular dystrophy, which may give rise to genuine stress incontinence, there is no simple genetic basis for urinary incontinence. However, a familial element may be present, especially in the case of detrusor instability and nocturnal enuresis. This is often the result of abnormal 'potty training', carried out by a parent with the condition, which leads to a reinforcement of abnormal behaviour patterns resulting in urinary symptoms.

'I'VE TRIED PELVIC FLOOR EXERCISES WHICH DIDN'T HELP'

Many women believe that their symptoms are due to weak pelvic floor muscles following childbirth. For women with detrusor instability this assumption is not valid, and pelvic floor exercises are of little benefit. Pelvic floor contractions are commonly taught to women following delivery, or when they complain of urinary incontinence. The belief is that pelvic floor training may prevent or even cure urinary incontinence. These exercises are usually carried out without supervision or vaginal examination, for example in an aerobics class, and are often incorrectly performed. There is little evidence to suggest that performing postnatal exercises protects against future incontinence. Even supervised Kegel exercises in women with proven genuine stress incontinence result in few complete cures. Most women will, however, derive a degree of symptomatic relief, and should be properly taught pelvic floor contractions with clear knowledge of their limitations.

'DRINKING PLENTY WILL HELP MY BLADDER PROBLEMS'

Unless symptoms are secondary to a urinary tract infection, increased fluid intake will only exacerbate symptoms of frequency, urgency, and incontinence. Excessive intake should be discouraged, but drastic reduction should also be avoided, especially in the elderly. We would usually recommend 1–1.5 l per day.

'I DON'T WANT TO END UP SMELLING OF URINE WHEN I'M OLD'

Urinary incontinence conjures up the image of an elderly woman surrounded by an ammoniacal odour. Even if the underlying problem cannot be cured, modern incontinence aids and appliances are available to help contain urinary leakage. Soiling of clothes should not occur with appropriate pads or pants. Correct medical and nursing management should ensure that the distress caused by urinary incontinence in the elderly is alleviated. Many women use sanitary towels, which are unsuitable and cause skin excoriation. Modern incontinence pads are expensive but can usually be provided free to women in the community, who should contact their local continence adviser for information.

'WILL I HAVE TO TAKE THESE TABLETS FOREVER?'

The treatment of detrusor instability is primarily pharmacological, using anticholinergic agents. Such drugs do not affect the underlying pathological process (often unknown) but merely provide symptomatic relief. Return of symptoms is usual upon cessation of treatment. It is common, however, to note spontaneous waxing and waning of the symptoms of detrusor instability, and therefore drug therapy may be reduced in times of remission. Since the therapeutic effect of most anticholinergic agents is paralleled by their side effects, patients should be encouraged to alter the dose of their medication to suit their needs. A dose reduction may be tried when side effects are troublesome, or when at home and in easy reach of the toilet. Conversely, increased dosage should be recommended to provide maximum cover, e.g. when out shopping or socializing. For oxybutynin this can be achieved relatively easily as it is a drug with a short half-life.

DELAY IN REFERRAL FOR INVESTIGATION OF URINARY INCONTINENCE

It is well documented that the number of women who present to their physician with urinary symptoms is small compared to the known prevalence of incontinence in the community. Some of the many reasons for delay in presentation volunteered by women attending our unit are shown below.

- Embarrassment or shame.
- Put up with minor disability.
- Insidious onset therefore lifestyle adapted to cope.
- Thought it was normal (many friends with same symptoms).
- Didn't think anything could be done to help.
- Thought it would go away.
- Fear of needing an operation.
- Heard that operations do no good.
- Didn't want to trouble doctors with trivial problems (denial of severity of disability).

Some women had in fact mentioned the problem to their general practitioner but were told that these problems are very common and will go away. Others were told to do pelvic floor exercises or given medication that did not help their symptoms.

Ignorance on the part of medical practitioners concerning the need for and the availability of incontinence services reinforces patients' misconceptions and contributes to delay in referral for investigation.

Many women only present once symptoms are severe and having a detrimental effect on their lifestyle. Common reasons for seeking medical advice are given below.

- Symptoms worsened (wearing pads all the time).
- Restricted social, work, family life.
- Incontinence during intercourse.
- Depression.
- Nocturnal symptoms (unable to sleep, bedwetting).
- Worried that symptoms will worsen when they get older.
- Unable to play sport/exercise.
- Unable to socialize/drink alcohol.

- Experienced a particularly embarrassing incident, e.g. leaked in public.
- Body image distortion/feelings of guilt and shame.
- Starting to smell.
- Marital problems.
- Have put up with it long enough.

Education of both lay public and medical personnel is essential to improve the standards of care for women with incontinence. Even though it is not always possible to cure the problem, symptoms can normally be alleviated with a subsequent improvement in quality of life.

11

Management of patients with the 'urge syndrome'

INTRODUCTION

The term 'urge syndrome' is used to describe a clinical condition which presents with a characteristic combination of urinary symptoms comprising urgency, urge incontinence, frequency, nocturia, and sometimes dysuria. Such symptoms are referred to as irritative and hence the label of an 'irritable bladder' is sometimes ascribed to these women.

Whilst implying a particular clinical picture, the term 'urge syndrome' is not a diagnosis. Each urinary symptom may occur alone, or in combination, and so the range of possible presentations and underlying diagnoses is wide. The condition may arise as a result of gynaecological, urological, medical, and even psychological pathology, so each patient must be assessed carefully in order to ensure appropriate management.

The presence of a urinary tract infection (UTI) may account for the symptoms of the urge syndrome, although actual incontinence is unusual. All women presenting with symptoms of lower urinary tract dysfunction should have a mid-stream specimen of urine (MSU) screened for infection, using microscopy, culture, and sensitivity. It is especially important to exclude a UTI if further tests involving catheterization or instrumentation of the lower urinary tract are contemplated. Women with recurrent UTIs should be differentiated from those with irritative symptoms due to other causes, by careful documentation of MSU results. In all genuine cases of recurrent UTI, intravesical pathology and voiding difficulties must be excluded by further investigation.

Any abdomino-pelvic mass can give rise to urinary symptoms, either due to restriction of bladder filling, or outflow obstruction. Thus frequency, urgency, bladder discomfort during filling, and voiding difficulty are all possible consequences. Not infrequently a woman with uterine fibroids or a large ovarian cyst presents with urinary symptoms. Similarly the increase in urinary symptoms in pregnancy is in part due to a pressure effect of the gravid uterus.

Careful abdominal and vaginal examination will detect significant masses which can give rise to urinary symptoms. Their presence may be confirmed by ultrasonography. It may be prudent, however, to carry out further investigations, including cystometry, prior to treatment. It is possible for a woman with uterine fibroids also to have lower urinary tract dysfunction, e.g. detrusor instability. In such a case, hysterectomy is unlikely to ameliorate all urinary symptoms.

Detrusor instability and sensory urgency are two common conditions that give rise to the symptoms of the urge syndrome. A detailed account of the investigation and management of detrusor instability is contained elsewhere in the book (see pp. 96–107).

SENSORY URGENCY

Definition   Sensory urgency, like detrusor instability is diagnosed following cystometry. There is no ICS definition, but the condition is characterized by painful catheterization, an early first sensation on bladder filling, and a reduced bladder capacity in the absence of detrusor instability.

Incidence   Exact figures are not known, but sensory urgency is a common finding in women with irritative symptoms of frequency, nocturia, urgency, and dysuria.

Increased bladder sensation

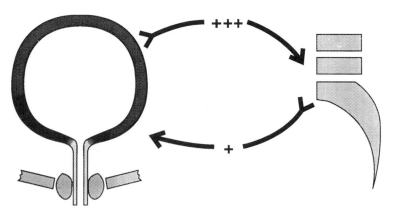

Fig. 11.1 Pathophysiology of sensory urgency.

Pathophysiology   See Fig. 11.1.

Clinical features   Mainly symptoms of frequency, urgency, and dysuria. Bladder may be tender on palpation.

Aetiology and associated factors   In most cases of sensory urgency, no underlying cause is found. Urine should be cultured for infection, and cystourethroscopy performed to exclude calculi and neoplasia. Bladder biopsy may be performed at the same time to exclude the possibility of interstitial cystitis (proliferation of mast cells within the detrusor muscle).
    The causes of sensory urgency are summarized below.

- Idiopathic.
- Urinary tract infection/inflammation.
- Bladder calculi.
- Interstitial cystitis.
- Transitional-cell carcinoma.

Treatment In all cases, an underlying condition should be sought and treated appropriately. Anticholinergic agents and bladder retraining are employed in the treatment of idiopathic sensory urgency. The treatment of interstitial cystitis is discussed below.

INTERSTITIAL CYSTITIS

In its most severe form interstitial cystitis is a painful, debilitating, ulcerative pancystitis, occurring predominantly in females (Hunner 1915). Its aetiology remains obscure, and treatment is often ineffective. Lower abdominal pain, perineal discomfort, dysuria, and dyspareunia are common findings in addition to irritative bladder symptoms. The presence of florid ulceration of the bladder mucosa on cystoscopy is characteristic, but a rare finding. The formation of petechial haemorrhages on refill cystoscopy may be seen in some milder cases of interstitial cystitis. Often, however, no objective abnormality is visible. Recently the presence of mast cells in the detrusor muscle has been used as a marker of the disease.

Up to a third of women with 'idiopathic sensory urgency' may be suffering from early interstitial cystitis (Frazer *et al.* 1990).

Treatment Interstitial cystitis may be treated using antihistamines, anticholinergic agents, oral steroids, or azathioprine. Surgical procedures including bladder distension, laser ablation of ulcers, enterocystoplasty, and cystectomy with urinary diversion have all been attempted, but should be reserved for women with severe, long-standing symptoms unresponsive to medical management.

High doses of oral prednisolone may be administered with good effect, and then reduced gradually after approximately three months treatment.

Intravesical instillation of dimethyl sulphoxide (DMSO) has been widely used in the treatment of interstitial cystitis, with symptomatic improvement rates of 50–90 per cent. A corresponding increase in bladder capacity is sometimes achieved together with clinical evidence of improvement in cystoscopic findings.

Sodium pentosanpolysulphate is a polyionic analogue of heparin, which enhances the glycosaminoglycan (GAG) mucus layer within the bladder. Given orally in a dose of 200–300 mg daily it has been shown to reduce symptoms of bladder pain, urgency, and nocturia in 80 per cent of 24 patients with interstitial cystitis. More recent studies, however, have not shown such efficacy, especially in the presence of ulcers.

A preliminary report of the use of intravesical doxorubicin showed marked symptomatic relief and healing of ulceration in three patients following weekly instillations for six weeks.

THE URETHRAL SYNDROME

This describes the association of frequency, urgency, and dysuria in the absence of significant bacteriuria. It is essentially a diagnosis of exclusion, once urinary tract infection, detrusor instability, sensory urgency, and local urethral pathology have been eliminated by careful investigation. It is more common in young nulliparous women.

In some cases, pyruria may be present in the absence of organisms, giving rise to the popular theory of infection with fastidious organisms such as *Chlamydia trachomatis*, *Ureaplasma urealyticum*, and *Mycoplasma hominis*. It is also possible that bacterial counts of 100 000/ml produce symptoms in certain women.

Other hypotheses regarding the aetiology of the urethral syndrome include urethral obstruction and spasm, post-menopausal hypoestrogenism, and psychogenic causes.

The evidence of outflow obstruction in these women is unconvincing, and so the use of urethral dilatation is seldom recommended. Similarly urethrotomy confers no benefit to women with the urethral syndrome unless there is proven outflow obstruction.

The urethra is supplied with oestrogen receptors and it is clear that oestrogen supplementation results in a reduction in irritative urinary symptoms in a proportion of post-menopausal women. Loss of vaginal lubrication will lead to increased urethral trauma and irritation following intercourse. This may be prevented by the application of vaginal lubricants and oestrogen therapy.

Psychological factors may play a role in some women with the urethral syndrome. On psychometric testing, such women score higher for anxiety, depression, dysphoria, hostility, and irritability than controls. Interpersonal problems are more common in women with the urethral syndrome, and the symptoms can be a means of avoiding sexual contact, consciously or unconsciously.

Cultures from the introitus, urethra, and bladder must be obtained. Urine cultures should be negative although pus cells may be seen on microscopy. Urine cytology should be negative for malignant cells. Cystourethroscopy is essentially normal, although evidence of inflammation of the urethra and trigone may be seen. Urodynamic investigation is normal, except in the few cases with associated urethral obstruction.

Treatment of the urethral syndrome

Increased fluid intake, in order to 'flush out' presumptive infectious organisms, will result in worse urinary frequency, and may exacerbate other symptoms. Perfumed soaps and douches should be avoided as they will only irritate the urethra further. The bladder should be emptied prior to and immediately following intercourse.

Alkalinizing agents may confer some relief from dysuria. In the presence of pyuria, it is reasonable to administer doxycycline or erythromycin in low dosage for two weeks, as an empirical treatment for chlamydial infection.

Urethral dilatation should only be performed in cases of proven outflow obstruction. If short-term symptomatic relief is achieved, then urethrotomy may be performed as its effects are longer lasting. Cryocautery of the urethra under local anaesthesia has been used, with good effect in a high proportion of cases. It probably has an effect by damaging the sensory nerves which supply the urethra.

Bladder retraining is often helpful to reduce troublesome frequency and urgency but is unlikely to affect dysuria or urethral discomfort.

REFERENCES

Frazer, M.I., Haylen, B.T., and Sissons, M. (1990). Do women with sensory urgency have early interstitial cystitis? *Br. J. Urol.*, **66**, 274–8.
Hunner, G.L. (1915). A rare type of bladder ulcer in women; report of cases. *Boston Med. Surg. J.*, **172**, 660–5.

12

Urinary tract infections

INTRODUCTION

Acute infection of the female urinary tract is common and has a multifactorial pathogenesis. It is generally considered that a pure growth of at least 10^5 organisms/ml obtained from a clean catch, mid-stream specimen of urine is indicative of infection (Kass 1957). It has been estimated that there are approximately one and a half million cases each year in the United Kingdom, and of these up to 25 per cent may go on to have recurrent infections. The occurrence of three or more episodes of urinary infection over a period of one year constitutes recurrent urinary tract infection. There is a double peak in the prevalence of this condition, one occurring in the 30–40 age group and the other between 55 and 65 years.

PATHOGENESIS

Microorganisms readily enter the bladder from the vagina and perineum, but are usually eliminated by complete voiding. Anything that impairs bladder emptying will predispose to urinary tract infection. Sexual intercourse and use of the contraceptive diaphragm are associated factors, but tampon usage is not associated with an increase in acute infection rates (if patients are controlled for sexual activity).

It is estimated that 13 per cent of women over 60 suffer with recurrent infections of the bladder and/or urethra. In institutionalized geriatric patients, this figure may well be much higher. The incidence of complications of acute UTI, such as pyelonephritis, is high in post-menopausal women, occurring in up to 30 per cent of cases. This increased incidence of recurrent UTIs in post-menopausal women may be related to the hypo-oestrogenic status or may be an age-related phenomenon.

INVESTIGATION

The degree and type of investigation required for patients with recurrent urinary infection is disputed. An MSU is mandatory and antibiotic therapy should be tailored to the results of culture and sensitivity tests. Intravenous urography is almost always normal and is not recommended as an initial outpatient investigation. Upper-tract pathology may be adequately investigated by renal ultrasound plus a plain X-ray showing kidneys, ureters, and bladder (KUB film) in all but a few cases.

Cystourethroscopy is commonly performed on patients with recurrent urinary infection. In our experience, few abnormalities other than those consistent with infection are detected. Morphological abnormalities can be diagnosed, however, and bladder-base biopsy may show evidence of chronic inflammation. Cystourethroscopy is more relevant in the elderly, since recurrent UTIs may be the presenting symptoms of a transitional-cell carcinoma.

Urodynamic investigation in women less than forty years old with recurrent UTIs is usually normal. Detrusor instability, giving rise to symptoms of the urge syndrome, and evidence of mechanical outflow obstruction are not common in this group (Burton and Cardozo, unpublished). Urodynamics is indicated, however, for women who have undergone previous bladder-neck surgery, of whom a high proportion will be shown to have mechanical outflow obstruction. Similarly in women who complain of persistent symptoms of 'cystitis', but with repeated negative urine cultures, the diagnostic yield from urodynamics is high. In this latter group, detrusor instability predominates, but voiding difficulties are also common.

TREATMENT OF RECURRENT UTI

General

Treatment should be aimed at the underlying condition which predisposes to recurrent infection. Incomplete bladder emptying should be adequately investigated urodynamically and treatment implemented to enhance bladder contractility using cholinergic agents, or to reduce urethral resistance pharmacologically or surgically where appropriate. Surgical repair of a cystourethrocele may improve voiding by 'unkinking' the urethra and lead to resolution of the problems of recurrent UTI. Constipation and faecal impaction are common causes of voiding difficulty in the elderly. They should be treated appropriately as they predispose to urinary tract infection.

Antibiotic therapy

Antibiotics are indicated for the treatment of acute urinary tract infection, but their role in management of women with recurrent UTI is limited. Long-term use of antibiotics is seldom indicated since the development of resistant bacterial strains may lead to increased morbidity. In particular, long-term prophylaxis should not be used in women with indwelling catheters as colonization of the lower tract will still occur, and morbidity is not altered. Alternatively, each infection should be managed individually with urine culture and appropriate therapy. Prophylactic antibiotics may be appropriate before intercourse if this is a closely associated factor.

The role of oestrogens

Lack of oestrogenic stimulation in post-menopausal women leads to a reduction in glycogen production by the vaginal epithelium. This results in loss of commensal organisms such as lactobacilli which require glycogen for metabolism. Vaginal pH rises and Gram-negative faecal organisms may colonize the vagina.

Atrophy of the vagina, urethra, and trigone predisposes to the ascent of infection into the bladder. Oestrogen supplementation improves the vaginal, urethral, and trigonal epithelium and leads to a restoration of the usual pre-menopausal vaginal flora. In this way it may be useful in the prevention of recurrent urinary tract infection.

REFERENCE

Kass, E.H. (1957). Bacteriuria and the diagnosis of infections of the urinary tract. *A.M.A. Arch. Int. Med.*, **100**, 709–14.

13

Congenital malformations

INTRODUCTION

Young girls may complain of diurnal or nocturnal incontinence. Detrusor instability may be present and represent delayed control over bladder function. Others may suffer with recurrent infections and a variable degree of incontinence when infected. A small number will have congenital anomalies which give rise to their symptoms. Stress incontinence is an uncommon finding in girls and suggests a congenital anomaly, such as epispadias. Similarly, true continual leakage is usually due to an anatomical defect, e.g. ectopic ureter.

INVESTIGATION

Physical examination is helpful as bladder exstrophy, epispadias, and urogenital sinus abnormalities can be identified. Further investigation by ultrasonography is indicated to exclude upper-tract duplication and is non-invasive. IVU is unpleasant and not required routinely. Urethroscopy is unhelpful except in urogenital sinus anomalies. Cystometry or videocystourethrography is useful in detecting neuropathic bladders but not routinely necessary for structural anomalies.

ECTOPIC URETERS

In duplex systems, the accessory ureteric bud fails to make contact with the urogenital sinus and enters the Müllerian system, resulting in incontinence. It may enter the vestibule, vagina, or, rarely, the uterus. Single ectopic ureters nearly always enter the urethra just below the level of the bladder neck.

The child presents with continual incontinence and otherwise normal voiding pattern. The ectopic opening can not usually be seen except on examination under anaesthesia. Renal function is often impaired and there is gross dilatation of the affected ureter. In cases of bilateral single ectopic ureters, the trigone is

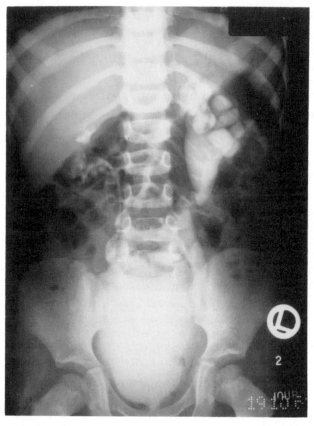

Fig. 13.1 An intravenous urogram demonstrating left-sided ectopic ureter with gross hydronephrosis.

absent and the bladder neck is incompetent. Reimplantation of the ureters and reconstruction of the bladder neck are required. In cases of duplex ureteric ectopia, the upper renal pole is usually dysplastic and should be excised together with the ectopic ureter. These abnormalities are extremely rare (Fig. 13.1).

UROGENITAL SINUS ABNORMALITIES

Several rare conditions exist in which the bladder and vagina share a common vulval orifice. Surgery is required to provide an adequate vaginal opening and to create a functioning bladder neck and urethra to provide urinary continence. Usually, however, a urinary diversion is required, or extensive reconstructive surgery.

EXSTROPHIC ABNORMALITIES

This occurs in 1 in 30 000 liveborn females, and arises due to failure of primitive streak mesoderm to invade the allantoic extension of the infra-umbilical mesoderm. The pelvic viscera are laid open on the surface of the abdomen with divergence of the recti and pubic bones. The urethra is open along its entire length, the clitoris is bifid and the labia widely separated.

Primary reconstruction should be attempted unless the bladder is too small to be usable. Results are improved if the bony pelvic defect can be closed, often necessitating osteotomy. Anti-reflux procedures and bladder-neck surgery should be delayed.

Long-term problems of reconstruction include continuing bladder-neck incompetence, persistent low bladder capacity due to low compliance, overflow incontinence, and upper tract obstruction, infection, and reflux. In a few cases urinary diversion is required.

EPISPADIAS

This is a less extensive defect resulting in a urethra with a deficient dorsal aspect and a bifid clitoris. The urethral sphincter is usually absent and the bladder neck incompetent so the child is incontinent. Ultrasonography to assess the upper tracts and cystometry to assess bladder capacity and compliance is preferable. Urethral repair and bladder-neck reconstruction are undertaken as for exstrophy but the results are superior.

SPINA BIFIDA

Fortunately, due to effective pre-natal diagnosis, this condition is much less common. In the past, associated urinary problems were dealt with by diversion, but nowadays reconstructive surgery, including the implantation of an artificial sphincter, is carried out.

14

The elderly

INTRODUCTION

The prevalence of urinary incontinence increases with age, and as many as 40 per cent of women in their eighties may be affected. The predominant cause of incontinence in this group is detrusor instability.

Medical disorders are common in the elderly, and may predispose to urinary incontinence. These age-associated disorders include senile dementia, cerebrovascular accident, Parkinsonism, spinal-cord disease, autonomic neuropathy, endocrine abnormalities, and urinary tract infections. Oestrogen deficiency results in atrophy of all layers of the bladder and urethra and may give rise to urinary symptoms.

Faecal impaction is a common cause of both voiding difficulty and overflow incontinence and should always be excluded. Decreased mobility and limited dexterity may also contribute to incontinence. In general, anything which reduces the independence of elderly women may result in temporary urinary incontinence, e.g. acute illness, hip fractures, and a change of environment such as hospitalization.

A full drug history is especially important since elderly patients are commonly prescribed diuretics, antidepressants, minor and major tranquillizers, all of which alter detrusor and urethral function.

Investigation of elderly patients need not always include full urodynamic investigation. A full clinical assessment, exclusion of a urinary tract infection, and the presence of a significant urinary residual by ultrasound may be all that is required prior to commencement of conservative treatment. A trial of anti-cholinergic therapy or bladder retraining will result in symptomatic improvement in a good proportion of patients. Only those patients who fail to respond need to be referred for further investigation, including urodynamic studies.

Since detrusor instability is the commonest cause of incontinence in this age group, subtracted cystometry may be used as a screening test with a high sensitivity for DI, which is less stressful for the patient than videocystourethrography. The number and complexity of investigations should be kept to a minimum whenever possible. Extra time should be allocated to allow for adequate investigation.

DETRUSOR INSTABILITY

The half-life of many drugs, including anticholinergics, is prolonged in the elderly. For this reason the smallest therapeutic dose should be employed and this should only be increased gradually to minimize side effects. Behavioural intervention in the form of bladder retraining is preferable, as it is efficacious with no side effects. Drugs and bladder drill are often needed together. Alternative treatments such as maximal electrical stimulation should be considered for those patients who fail or cannot tolerate drug therapy.

GENUINE STRESS INCONTINENCE

Surgery remains the primary mode of treatment for this condition, although conservative measures should be considered in those with mild symptoms and in those unfit for surgery.

Oestrogen replacement in combination with an α-agonist (e.g. phenylpropanolamine) may reduce incontinence in a proportion of women (Hilton *et al.* 1990).

Pelvic floor exercises and other forms of pelvic floor re-education may be used but tend to be less effective than in younger women.

The choice of surgical procedure employed may be affected by several factors. Atrophy of the vulva and vagina or previous vaginal surgery may result in limited mobility of the vaginal tissues, such that a colposuspension is not possible. A minority of patients may be unfit for major abdominal surgery with a relatively long anaesthetic time. In either case, an endoscopic bladder-neck suspension such as the Stamey procedure is employed. Anaesthetic time is reduced, less vaginal mobility is required, and success rates are comparable to those of the colposuspension, at least in the short term. The efficacy of paraurethral collagen injections is currently being evaluated, and may prove to be of benefit in the elderly or in women who have undergone multiple previous incontinence operations.

VOIDING DIFFICULTIES

The presence of a urinary residual may indicate detrusor underactivity or outflow obstruction due to a urethral stricture, faecal impaction, or a pelvic mass. In cases of severe voiding difficulties, overflow incontinence may result. Faecal impaction should be treated aggressively with suppositories and enemas. Voiding cystometry and urethral pressure profilometry will distinguish between an underactive detrusor or outflow obstruction. Proven urethral stricture should be treated surgically by urethral dilatation or urethrotomy, whereas detrusor underactivity may be treated medically using cholinergic agents or more commonly by intermittent self-catheterization. If the latter is not possible due to poor vision or limited dexterity, an indwelling catheter, either suprapubic or urethral may be appropriate.

AIDS AND EQUIPMENT

Many aids are available which make life easier for elderly patients and promote continence. Commodes may be used in the home where access to the toilet is difficult, e.g. when it is upstairs or outside. Raised toilet seats and grab rails may be fitted to existing toilets to make them easier and safer to use. Advice regarding suitable clothing should be given. Garments should be washable and easy to remove quickly prior to micturition. This is especially important for women with poor manual dexterity or urge incontinence. Pads and pants are available in many different forms and may be obtained free of charge from district nurses or the district continence advisor. This is discussed further in Chapter 17.

REFERENCE

Hilton, P., Tweddell, A.L., and Mayne, C. (1990). Oral and intravaginal estrogens alone and in combination with alpha-adrenergic stimulation in genuine stress incontinence. *Int. Urogynecol. J.*, **1**, 80–6.

15

Pregnancy

INTRODUCTION

Pregnancy is a time when many bodily functions undergo change and the lower urinary tract is no exception. Anatomical changes take place due to the enlarged uterus which initially forms a space-occupying lesion in the pelvis and, later on, an abdominal mass. There are marked changes in hormone levels and of particular relevance are the raised levels of progesterone and oestrogen which occur. In addition, labour and delivery may result in trauma to the pelvic floor.

The upper urinary tract is also affected by pregnancy. Under normal circumstances, the bladder fills at a rate of 60 ml/h from the kidneys, via the ureters. During pregnancy the glomerular filtration rate is increased and there is evidence of ureteric dilatation in up to 90 per cent of women.

SYMPTOMS

Lower urinary tract symptoms are very common in pregnancy. It was originally believed that diurnal frequency is worst in early pregnancy but thereafter gradually improves. This, however, is not now considered to be true. Once frequency develops it tends not to get better but rather deteriorates towards term (Francis 1961).

There is much debate as to whether it is pregnancy itself or labour which results in stress incontinence. Although there have been several retrospective and a few prospective studies looking at this subject, it is important to appreciate that stress incontinence is merely a symptom and not synonymous with urethral sphincter incompetence.

Stress incontinence normally occurs for the first time in the antenatal period and once present deteriorates towards term (Stanton *et al.* 1980). It has been suggested that most cases of stress incontinence are reversible, with only a minority remaining incontinent in the long term, and that very few cases originate following delivery.

In addition, urgency, urge incontinence, and symptoms of voiding difficulties have been shown to be fairly common in pregnancy but subsequently resolve post-partum.

CAUSES OF INCONTINENCE

Distortion of the fundus of the bladder by the enlarged uterus was thought to be the cause of urinary frequency. It is more likely that frequency is due to increased urine output in pregnancy and nocturia may be due to increased urine production, decreased bladder capacity, and increased hours spent in bed.

Recently we have demonstrated that pregnancy results in an increased prevalence of detrusor instability which resolves postnatally. Although this may explain the high prevalence of incontinence antenatally, we found little correlation between symptoms and urodynamics in pregnancy (Cutner *et al.* 1991).

It is suggested that changes in the position of the bladder neck during labour results in stretching of supporting structures which leads to damage and weakening of the urethral sphincter mechanisms. Indeed, pregnant fascia has a reduced tensile strength which may account for the development of stress incontinence in pregnancy. Although post-partum the fascia will regain its previous strength, it may be that in cases of permanent stress incontinence it has already undergone irreversible damage by over-stretching.

Studies have demonstrated significantly reduced urethral pressure profile parameters in post-partum primiparous women who had undergone vaginal delivery when compared with normal nulliparous controls. In addition, pelvic floor denervation occurs in women having a vaginal delivery but not those undergoing Caesarean section.

A long first stage and a long active (pushing) second stage have both been shown to result in urethral damage. It has been suggested that epidural analgesia affords protection to the pelvic floor during delivery by enabling relaxation during delivery.

The association between delivery factors and stress incontinence postnatally does not explain the high prevalence of this symptom antenatally. It may be that the symptom is due to different causes in the antenatal period, possibly detrusor instability. However, it has been suggested that stress incontinence antenatally is physiological, with most cases resolving after delivery. If this were the case it would be important to identify those women who are susceptible to development of permanent stress incontinence if allowed a vaginal delivery in order that a prophylactic Caesarean section might be undertaken.

REFERENCES

Cutner, A., Cardozo, L.D., and Benness, C.J. (1991). Assessment of urinary symptoms in early pregnancy. *Br. J. Obstet. Gynaecol.*, **98**, 1283–6.

Francis, W.J.A. (1961). Disturbances of bladder function in relation to pregnancy. *J. Obstet. Gynaecol. Br. Empire*, **67**, 353–65.

Stanton, S.L., Kerr-Wilson, R., and Harris, G.V. (1980). The incidence of urological symptoms in normal pregnancy. *Br. J. Obstet. Gynaecol.*, **87**, 897–900.

16

Mixed incontinence

INTRODUCTION

The treatment of each condition has been addressed in turn. However, it is not uncommon for more than one abnormality to be present. Although it is normal for one type of dysfunction to be the main complaint, the other may jeopardize effective treatment.

GENUINE STRESS INCONTINENCE AND DETRUSOR INSTABILITY

It is always difficult to know what to do when stress and urge incontinence coexist. Should genuine stress incontinence or detrusor instability be treated first (Karram and Bhatia 1989)? We would recommend conservative management in the first instance. This should be with anticholinergic agents for the detrusor instability and some form of pelvic floor exercises for the genuine stress incontinence. If the woman is post-menopausal, hormone replacement therapy should be instituted as this is of benefit to both conditions. Some women will be cured by this combination of treatment.

If the woman still complains of incontinence, then urodynamic investigations should be repeated whilst on drug treatment. If genuine stress incontinence is diagnosed then operative treatment for genuine stress incontinence is indicated but the patient must be warned that it may aggravate her irritative bladder symptoms. Obviously if detrusor instability is still present, then further management of this condition is indicated and an incontinence operation should not be carried out as the symptoms of urgency and frequency may be exacerbated.

GENUINE STRESS INCONTINENCE AND VOIDING DIFFICULTIES

Operations for genuine stress incontinence will aggravate any underlying voiding difficulties, by increasing outflow obstruction. These women are best treated initially with pelvic floor exercises but if this is unsuccessful an operation will be necessary.

Such a patient undergoing an operative procedure should be warned of the possibility of voiding problems post-operatively. If voiding difficulties are pronounced pre-operatively, then she should be taught clean intermittent self-catheterization prior to the operation to confirm that she is happy that continence, at the expense of the need to do this indefinitely, is a satisfactory solution.

DETRUSOR INSTABILITY AND VOIDING DIFFICULTIES

Detrusor instability is normally treated with anticholinergic agents. However, these will compromise detrusor function and aggravate voiding difficulties. They may precipitate urinary retention in a susceptible patient.

If the voiding difficulties are mild, detrusor instability may be treated with bladder drill or anticholinergic agents but urinary residuals must be monitored. A chronic urinary residual, however, may be the cause of urinary frequency and can even result in detrusor instability. Paradoxically such women may be cured of both pathologies by cholinergic agents.

Where the voiding difficulties are not due to urethral obstruction but rather poor detrusor function, it may be necessary to treat with anticholinergic agents in combination with clean intermittent self-catheterization. These women should measure their urinary residual as, with time, the need for catheterization may become unnecessary.

If the voiding difficulties are due to urethral outflow obstruction, a urethrotomy in combination with anticholinergic agents may treat both conditions. It is advisable to fully investigate these women prior to urethrotomy as the high urethral pressure could be the sole reason why leakage does not occur with each detrusor contraction and a urethrotomy may precipitate urinary incontinence.

REFERENCE

Karram, M.M. and Bhatia, N.N. (1989). Management of coexistent stress and urge urinary incontinence. *Obstet. Gynecol.*, **73**, 4–7.

17

Pads, pants, and appliances

INTRODUCTION

Incontinence aids and appliances are not traditionally the province of the general practitioner. However, general practitioners and practice nurses may be asked for information and advice about incontinence aids.

The range of products available is extensive, so a working knowledge of what can be prescribed can be of enormous value. Different incontinence aids are available within each district, but the choice of products that can be purchased privately is greater. This may unfortunately lead to inappropriate use of certain products and unnecessary expense.

Often, incontinence aids are prescribed or bought as a last resort. They help to deal with the problem but will not cure it. It is important that incontinence should first be investigated, and the underlying condition treated. In this way, the need for aids may be avoided or modified. Requirements may change with ongoing treatment, or with the passage of time.

Before any aids can be prescribed or allocated, a full assessment of that patients needs will be required to ensure optimal benefit. This would generally take the form of a nursing assessment carried out in the patients own home by a district nurse or continence adviser. Important points to consider would include the following.

1. Degree and type of incontinence.
2. Lifestyle of patient, i.e. employment, social activities, personal relationships.

3. Mobility and dexterity.
4. Layout of dwelling including provision of toilet facilities.
5. Is a carer available?
6. Concurrent medication.
7. Fluid balance.

Pads and pants cannot be prescribed by a general practitioner, these are provided through the Health Authority via the district nurses and continence advisory services. Other aids (catheters and leg bags) can be prescribed.

PADS AND PANTS

Pants

There are several types of pants available on the market which can be adapted to suit most degrees of incontinence (Fig. 17.1).

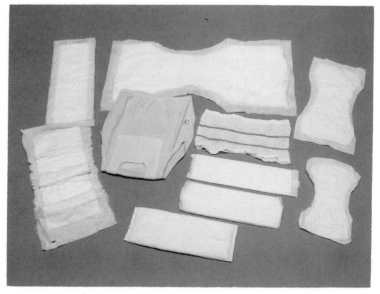

Fig. 17.1 A selection of incontinence pads and pants.

Stretch pants

These are the most lightweight and are made of washable nylon net. They can be worn with a wide range of plastic-backed pads, and are close fitting and cheap. They can be used for light to heavy incontinence and night-time incontinence.

Marsupial pants

As the name suggest, these are manufactured from a one-way fabric with a special pouch into which a pad can be fitted, thereby keeping plastic away from the skin. They have the advantage of allowing the wearer to change the pads without changing pants. This type of garment should be well fitted and is available in many styles, but is not suitable for heavy urinary incontinence or double incontinence. Any pants with a plastic gusset should not be used with plastic-backed pads as double layers of plastic will encourage skin irritation and chafing. The main disadvantage is that the soiled pouch remains in contact with the skin when the pad is changed.

Waterproof pants

These are still available through many outlets, but many continence advisers do not recommend their use. They are generally made from a soft PVC with a nylon pouch into which is placed a non-plastic-backed pad. The main drawback is that damage to skin is caused through chafing, leading to irritation and local infection. This is similar to nappy rash.

Washable pants

Washable pants have a special absorbent gusset which will absorb urine and can be washed in the normal way. These types of pads and pants are only helpful for light incontinence.

Pads

Pads are manufactured in numerous shapes and sizes. They are designed for heavy use, for example during the night, through to light daytime incontinence. The Health Authority will only provide certain products which have proven efficacy and are cost effective. The supply of pads is under the jurisdiction of the continence adviser and district nursing service. The products used in hospital may vary from those supplied to the community. Supplies to nursing homes are provided by local social services whilst private nursing homes will supply their own.

Pads are essentially absorbent, body-worn rectangles. Recently the shape and absorbency of pads has been researched in an effort to find the most effective 'user-friendly' pad, but their general purpose remains the same (Fig. 17.1).

Absorbent roll

Not used as frequently as pads, they are made from cellulose with cotton-wool facings and a net cover. Pieces are cut from the roll as required, and are used with lightweight pants or normal underwear. Absorbent roll is only really useful for light incontinence.

Plastic-backed pads

Again these pads are manufactured in many shapes and absorbencies. They have a protective plastic backing and are for use with stretch pants, mesh pants, or normal underwear. They should not be used with any plastic or plastic-gusseted pants. They have a self-adhesive strip which will hold the pad in place.

Pouch pads

These are non-plastic-backed pads which can cope with different types of urinary incontinence depending on size and absorbency. These pads are designed to be used with the marsupial pants thus avoiding the double plastic layers.

Washable pads

Some pads are reusable and are made of a special polyester with waterproof backing which will absorb urine. These can be worn under normal underwear or stretch pants.

All-in-one pads

These are similar in form to babies' nappies and are worn without additional pants. They are particularly useful for heavy incontinence and are disposable. They are useful in cases of double incontinence.

Female body-worn appliances

Female anatomy does not lend itself well to body-worn devices. It is hard to create a leak-proof seal and the appliances are difficult to manage for less dextrous patients. The female urinary pouch is attached to the vulva with adhesive and is attached to a drainage bag. These pouches are not of great use in the community but can be used for women who need intensive nursing care. They are not available on prescription.

CATHETERS

Indwelling catheters are prescribed by the general practitioner usually on the advice of the continence adviser or district nurse. The patient needs to be assessed to decide which type of catheter should be used. This depends upon the sex of the patient and the duration of catheterization required. Shorter catheters are available for female use. Short-term catheters are made from Teflon-coated latex. Silicone, silicone elastomer, or hydrogel catheters are best suited for longer use (up to three months) after which they should be changed (Fig. 17.2).

The gauge of the catheter for routine drainage should be no more than 12 to 14 French gauge and the balloon should be filled to a maximum of 10 ml. This prevents damage to the sphincter, and reduces the risk of urinary infection and catheter bypassing due to detrusor instability.

Intermittent self-catheterization

Intermittent self-catheterization is an alternative to long-term indwelling catheterization in the manually dextrous. This is a method which must be taught by a suitably qualified health

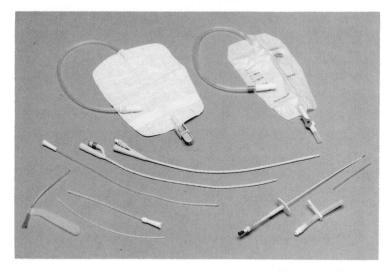

Fig. 17.2 A selection of urinary catheters (urethral and suprapubic) and two collecting bags designed to be worn on the leg.

professional but again the catheters are prescribed through the general practitioner.

LEG BAGS

These are designed to hold varying volumes of urine and have a capacity of 350 ml, 500 ml, or 750 ml. Outlet taps are designed to suit all types of manual ability and will allow direct connection to a larger bag for night drainage withought disconnecting the catheter. The bags can be body worn, being attached to a waist belt, or thigh or leg support straps. Women tend to wear thigh bags whilst men use calf leg bags. The main aim is to achieve discreet comfort and to avoid pulling and kinking of the catheter and tubing.

BED PROTECTION

Most appliances can be worn in bed, but leakage may occur. Beds can be protected by some form of plastic sheeting. This may be uncomfortable and may cause excessive sweating. Bed pads are usually made from layers of absorbent wadding with a plastic backing, are available in different sizes, and are disposable. Reusable bed pads are washable and are made from quilted absorbent material. The urine is absorbed through the one-way fabric, keeping the skin dry. This type of bed pad is manufactured in many different forms and availability varies from district to district.

OTHER AIDS

There are numerous aids available apart from the pads, pants, and appliances discussed above. These include the following.

1. Urinals, i.e. male or female receptacles.
2. Specially adapted clothing (to facilitate catheter management).
3. Drainage-bag stands.
4. Aids in the lavatory, e.g. raised lavatory seat, grab rails.
5. Commodes, sani-chairs, chemical toilets.

Adaptations to the home are the responsibility of the social services and occupational health workers.

A comprehensive list of aids and appliances is available in the Directory of continence aids and toileting aids, which is available from the Association for Continence Advice, which may be contacted through the Disabled Living Foundation (see p. 160).

Further reading on incontinence aids and their uses can be obtained from the list of addresses given below. The major pharmaceutical companies also offer help lines to advise sufferers. Most of their products are widely publicized. For the general practitioner the best sources of information are the continence advisory services and the district nursing services. They are able to give comprehensive advice on what is available to your patients, but more importantly which patients would most benefit from the resources available.

18

Failures

INTRODUCTION

In some women it may not be possible to cure incontinence. However, careful assessment of these women will nearly always facilitate an improvement in their quality of life. The different options available are shown in Table 18.1.

Table 18.1 Options available in the advent of failure to cure incontinence

Continence aids (Chapter 17)	Pads
	Pants
Permanent catheterization	Urethral
	Suprapubic
Urinary diversion	Ileal conduit
	Uretero-colic anastomosis
	Continent diversion

PERMANENT CATHETERIZATION

Some women find that the use of incontinence pads leads to skin excoriation and is associated with an unpleasant ammoniacal smell. The leakage of urine may be in large quantities or they may be physically handicapped such that coping with pads results in being continously wet. In addition, in some cases of voiding difficulties, the woman may not have sufficient manual dexterity to cope with clean intermittent self-catheterization. For these women a permanent indwelling catheter may be the best solution.

A urethral catheter is normally used. It is important that the smallest possible catheter is used. It should be silicone-coated and changed every three to six months. Sometimes even with a permanent indwelling catheter the woman remains wet as urine bypasses the catheter. This can be due to blockage of the catheter from debis in the bladder, or due to detrusor instability. Bypassing of the catheter is often treated by using a larger catheter with a balloon of greater volume. This is totally wrong as the urine will still bypass the catheter and detrusor instability will be worsened. In addition, the urethra will become a rigid large-bore tube such that urine continually bypasses.

If the woman starts to experience bypass of the catheter the solution is to reduce the size of both catheter and balloon, check for urinary tract infection, and to investigate for evidence of detrusor instability and bladder debris. Detrusor instability may require anticholinergic therapy, oral or intravesical (Ekstrom *et al.* 1990) and bladder debris is treated by regular bladder washouts. Sometimes changing the pH of the urine will prevent the formation of debris. If the patient has repeated urinary tract infections, long-term treatment with regular bladder washouts with a urinary antiseptic is preferable to continuous antibiotics, as otherwise resistance to organisms will develop.

Sometimes the urethra is of such large bore that a urethral catheter is unable to keep the woman dry. A solution is to occlude the urethra and to insert a permanent suprapubic catheter. This should be a silicone-coated Foley catheter managed in the same way as a urethral catheter.

URINARY DIVERSION

For those women in whom all else has failed or those with neuropathic disease, urinary diversion is sometimes the answer. Until recently an ileal conduit or uretero-colic anastomosis was employed. The former has the problem that the woman must wear a collecting bag continuously and the latter may result in electrolyte imbalance and faecal incontinence.

Nowadays continent diversions are undergoing evaluation. The patient has a continent nipple on the skin's surface which she catheterizes at regular intervals. The complications of such procedures are related to the type of diversion employed. The benefits of continent diversions are underoing evaluation and would appear to be promising.

SUMMARY

Although incontinence is not a life-threatening condition, it undoubtedly causes a great deal of patient morbidity. Most women can be cured, and the use of appropriate investigations prior to treatment will reduce the number of failures. In all cases, the quality of life of women with lower urinary tract dysfunction can be greatly improved.

REFERENCE

Ekstrom, B., Andersson, K.-E., and Mattiasson, A. (1990). Intravesical administration of drugs in patients with detrusor hyperactivity. *Neurourol. Urodyn.*, **9**, 16.

Appendix

Normal values

The International Continence Society has produced six reports on the terminology of lower urinary tract dysfunction. The first five have been incorporated into one collated report (Abrams *et al.* 1990). Only common terms and ranges of normal values necessary in the understanding of lower urinary tract function will be presented. Those definitions and normal values that are in common usage but are not defined by these reports are printed in bold type.

DEFINITIONS

Urinary incontinence is the involuntary loss of urine which is objectively demonstrable and is a social or hygienic problem.

Diurnal frequency: seven or more day-time voids.

Nocturia: two or more night-time voids.

Urge incontinence: the involuntary loss of urine associated with a strong desire to void (urgency).

Enuresis: any involuntary loss of urine.

Nocturnal enuresis: incontinence during sleep.

Dysuria: painful micturition.

Stress incontinence: symptom—complaining of the involuntary loss of urine during physical exertion. Sign—the observation of loss of urine synchronous with physical exertion.

SUBTRACTED CYSTOMETRY

Intravesical pressure: the pressure within the bladder.

Abdominal pressure: estimated from the rectal (vaginal) pressure.

Detrusor pressure: estimated by subtracting abdominal pressure from intravesical pressure.

CLASSIFICATION OF INCONTINENCE

Genuine stress incontinence: the involuntary loss of urine occurring when, in the absence of a detrusor contraction, the intravesical pressure exceeds the maximum urethral pressure.

Unstable detrusor (phasic detrusor contractions): one which is shown to objectively contract, spontaneously or on provocation, during the filling phase while the patient is attempting to inhibit micturition.

Low compliance: a rise in detrusor pressure of at least 10 cm H_2O for a filled volume of 300 ml or a rise of at least 15 cm H_2O for a filled volume of 500 ml.

Detrusor hyperreflexia: detrusor overactivity due to a disturbance of the nervous control mechanisms.

Sensory urgency: a reduced first sensation and bladder capacity associated with a strong desire to void and often painful catheterization.

Overflow incontinence: any involuntary loss of urine associated with over-distension of the bladder.

NORMAL VALUES

Normal fluid intake: between one and two litres per 24 h.

Positive pad test: in a one-hour pad test, a weight gain of more than 1 g is taken to signify incontinence. **Commonly 1.5 g is taken as the upper limit of normal.**

Peak flow rate: should be at least 15 ml/s for a volume voided of at least 150 ml.

Normal urinary residual: less than 50 ml.

Normal first sensation: 150–250 ml.

Normal maximum cystometric capacity: 400–600 ml.

Detrusor pressure rise on filling: less than 10 cm H_2O for 300 ml or 15 cm H_2O for 500 ml.

Maximum detrusor pressure during voiding: less than 60 cm H_2O.

Urethral pressure profilometry: no normal values defined.

REFERENCE

Abrams, P., Blaivas, J.G., Stanton, S.L., and Andersen, J.T. (1990). The standardisation of terminology of lower urinary tract function. *Br. J. Obstet. Gynaecol.* (Suppl.), **6**, 1–16.

Suggested further reading

Abrams, P., Fenely, R., and Torrens, M. (1983). *Urodynamics.* Springer, London.

Drife, J., Hilton, P., and Stanton, S.L. (1990). *Micturition.* Springer, London.

Freeman, R. and Malvern, J. (1989). *The unstable bladder.* John Wright, New York.

Jarvis, G.J. (1990). *Female urinary incontinence.* Royal College of Obstetricians and Gynaecologists, London.

Norton, P. (1990). *Urinary incontinence.* (Clinical Obstetrics and Gynaecology, vol. 33). Lippincott, USA.

Ostergard, D. and Bent, A. (1991). *Urogynaecology and urodynamics: theory and practice* (3rd edn). Williams and Wilkins, USA.

Stanton, S.L. (1992). *Clinical urogynaecology* (2nd edn). Churchill Livingstone, London. (In press.)

Stanton, S.L. and Tanagho, E. (1986). *Surgery of female incontinence* (2nd edn). Springer, Heidelberg.

Sutherst, J., Frazer, M., Richmond, D., and Haylen, B. (1990). *Introduction to clinical gynaecological urology.* Butterworth-Heinemann, London.

Useful addresses

Association for Continence Advice
contact through the Disabled Living Foundation.

Disabled Living Foundation
Incontinence Advisory Service,
380–384 Harrow Road,
London,
W9 2HU.
Tel. 071 266 3704.

Disabled Living Centre
Orthotic and Aids Service,
Musgrave Park Hospital,
Stockmans Lane,
Belfast,
BT9 7JB.
Tel. 0232 669501.

The Demonstration Aids Centre
The Lodge,
Rookwood Hospital,
Llandaff,
Cardiff,
Mid Glamorgan,
CF5 2YN.
Tel. 0222 566281 x5166.

Disabled Living Centre
Astley Ainslie Hospital,
Grange Loan,
Edinburgh,
EH9 2HL.
Tel. 031 447 6271 x5653.

Disabled Living Services
Disabled Living Centre,
Redbank House,
4 St Chads Street,
Cheetham,
Manchester,
M8 8QA.
Tel. 061 832 3678.

Newcastle upon Tyne Council for the Disabled
The Dene Centre,
Castles Farm Road,
Newcastle upon Tyne,
NE3 1PH.
Tel. 091 284 0480.

Southampton Aid and Equipment Centre
Southampton General Hospital,
Tremona Road,
Southampton,
SO9 4XY.
Tel. 0703 777222 x3414.

Age Concern England
Asral House,
1268 London Road,
London,
SW16 4ER.
Tel. 081 679 8000.

National Action on Incontinence (consumer self-help group)
4 St Pancras Way,
London,
NW1 0PE.

Continence Advisory Service
National manned helpline 2–7p.m.
Tel. 091 213 0050.

British Association of Continence Carers
Helpline Tel. 0753 656716.

Continence Foundation
contact through the Disabled Living Foundation

Index